FROM
WATTS
TO THE
W🌍RLD

A CHRONICLE OF SERVICE

ROSALYN CAIN KING

FROM

WATTS

TO THE

W🌍RLD

When people hear about certain aspects of my career, I'm inevitably asked, "What did you do?" When they learn that I was a pharmacist, yet I traveled the world extensively working on global health issues, they often wonder how I could have spent so much time on the frontlines of public health rather than standing behind a counter dispensing medication. The truth is, I've done both of these things, and my career is a testament to the many ways that a pharmacist can contribute to the world of health care in general, and public health in particular, on both the local and global fronts.

I'm writing to set forth an account of events, to chronicle what I've been blessed to do all these years – what I did, where I did it, and why I was moved to follow the unique career path that I did. This book covers the highlights of my career and chronicles activities undertaken without deep analysis of those events. It is not intended to be an autobiography or a full account of my life, but rather an overview. It is designed to give the public health and pharmacist practitioner a wider view of pharmacy practice. It presents a record of professional actions in service to the underserved.

In the past, pharmacists were trained either to work in hospitals, community pharmacies, industrial settings, or academia. However, whenever medications are being discussed, pharmacists can have a seat at the table. They can contribute – whether it is in the context of policy, diplomacy, international health, or basic primary health care. But they have to show others at the table how those skills can be applied because other health professionals and policy makers may not understand that yet.

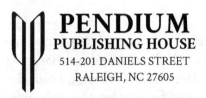

PENDIUM
PUBLISHING HOUSE
514-201 DANIELS STREET
RALEIGH, NC 27605

Dedication

This book is dedicated to my mother, Ethel C. Davis, who was an encourager of excellence, a stalwart pioneer in data processing, and a woman who introduced the idea of computing to me even before the technology was widely known.

She was one of the first Black keypunch operators for the federal government in the early 1940s, and when she retired in 1979, she was the head of the data processing branch for the entire eastern region of the Federal Aviation Administration.

But that was only one side of my mother. She was also a faithful community leader and membership chair of the Hempstead, NY chapter of the National Association for the Advancement of Colored People. In fact, we recently dedicated a brick to her memory at the National Civil Rights Museum in Memphis, Tennessee.

My mother coined the term 'stick-to-it-ive-ness.' While the phrase won't be found in anybody's dictionary, everybody knows exactly what it means. Once you start a task, you stick with it, and that's what my mother instilled in me.

She taught me that what you put in your mind, others could never strip from you – and in those days of heightened segregation, there was little else that the system could not take.

My mother was a pioneer in every sense of the word. She gave me the courage to lead.

This book is also dedicated to my gallant and gutsy spiritual-soulmate husband Sterling, a Son of the South, and my children: the late Kristin, our angel in Heaven, and Aaron Christopher, husband of Tina Falika King, and father of Sterling Richard and Aaryn Camille. To God be the Glory!

Contents

Foreword

I have prepared numerous book forewords during my career, but none of those dealt with a person as accomplished as Rosalyn King. It is difficult to know where to begin. There are many autobiographies written and published every year by people we may or may not have heard of who held high positions in government, academia, or in the private sector. Most of those persons did an adequate job but have little to claim in accomplishments other than holding on to their jobs for some period of time. In the following pages, we learn about a person who never chose to hold a high position and was never famous, but whose achievements dwarf most leaders in quality, quantity, and scope.

Rosalyn King is unique. She is a Black female pharmacist from a humble family who proved herself in the academic world, within the professional societies surrounding her areas of specialization, and in the U.S. government, as well as in international N.G.O.s and international agencies. I have known her for nearly fifty years and never tire of learning about her spectacular, usually pioneering, accomplishments. None of her accomplishments surprise me. To know her is to recognize that here is a person who cares about her fellow man first and foremost. Her early work (1970) on the Pharmacy and the Poor project for the American Pharmacists Association brought to light evidence of unacceptable disparities according to race and wealth. But unlike most studies, her work went on with suggested solutions and proposed remedies.

The following pages describe a career with more accomplishments than would be found by five ordinary persons. Her skin color probably was responsible for some resistance to her work, but it never stopped her, nor did her gender, both uncommon in the mid-to-late 20th century. This foreword will not spoil the reader's thrill of learning about the numerous phases of her career, each one successfully tackling ever more difficult and complex problems on four continents. Perhaps her own words provide a clue to what makes her tick: "Letting your difference make a difference."

It would be a fair and honest statement to say that her work has helped the quality of life in scores of countries, upgraded the level of science-based pharmacy education, and helped make the pharmacist be seen as a member of the health team and not merely as a seller of medical products. Roz King has boosted the careers of countless people and has served as a role model for many times that number of future pharmacists. She has worked tirelessly to incorporate public health principles and techniques into the pharmacy curriculum while personally demonstrating that her suggestions actually work, having been evaluated by her somewhere in the world. This publication could have been called: "Do as I do, not do as I say." Expect to be exhausted just by reading about her activities, one after the next; yet, that is Rosalyn King. I know the reader will be honored to learn about her, even if they do not ever have the honor of meeting her in person.

Albert I Wertheimer, PhD, MBA
Professor, Nova Southeastern University
Ft. Lauderdale, FL

Acknowledgements

This work would not have been possible without the support of so many who have played an integral role in my life. Some of them were instrumental in helping me to put my thoughts together to create this Chronicle of events in my career. Others had a profound effect on my life throughout my personal and professional journeys.

After acknowledging my help from God, I'd like to thank my husband Sterling, my guiding light.

I'd also like to acknowledge the legacy of the Handy family of Savannah, Georgia, which filled me with confidence and pride, and gave me my foundation.

I am especially grateful for my deep thinkers, my son Aaron and his wife Tina.

I'd also like to thank all of my early school friends who crossed my path from 8th grade at All Saints Grammar School, to Cathedral High School (All Saints Branch), and Hempstead High School in Hempstead, NY.

It's also important that I acknowledge all my past and current colleagues and collaborators. In particular, I'd like to thank those at Howard University Continuing Education and all those who were part of my work in Romania and Nigeria.

It is an honor to be recognized by the pharmacist, Dr. Albert Wertheimer, the Laureate for the 1998 Scheele Award in Sweden, which some say is the pharmacy equivalent of the Nobel Prize, and the 2019 Donald E. Francke Medal from the American Society of Health-System Pharmacists.

Finally, I'd like to thank all the students and practitioners who asked me what I did. This chronicle is for you – not as a roadmap, but as an example of how you must take risks to leave your footprints on the world.

Preface

When people hear about certain aspects of my career, I'm inevitably asked, "What did you do?" When they learn that I was a pharmacist, yet I traveled the world extensively working on global health issues, they often wonder how I could have spent so much time on the frontlines of public health rather than standing behind a counter dispensing medication. The truth is, I've done both of these things, and my career is a testament to the many ways that a pharmacist can contribute to the world of health care in general, and public health in particular, on both the local and global fronts.

An additional spark for this book was a chapter I wrote for the American Pharmacists Association on being a pharmacist, which was titled, "From Watts to the World: One Pharmacist's Journey," in 2010. Now I am writing this first-person narrative to set forth an account of events to chronicle what I've been blessed to do all these years – what I did, where I did it, and why I was moved to follow the unique career path that I did.

This book covers the highlights of my career and chronicles activities undertaken, without deep analysis of those events. It is not intended to be an autobiography or a full account of my life, but rather an overview. It is designed to give the public health and pharmacist practitioner a wider view of pharmacy practice. It presents a record of professional actions in service to the underserved.

Why is it important for me to tell this story now? Recently, I was elected to the National Pharmaceutical Association Foundation Board. I was nominated and named a Fellow of the National Pharmaceutical Association, a lifetime appointment. I was also appointed the National Pharmaceutical Association Foundation representative to the National Pharmaceutical Association Board of Directors. Those activities compel me to answer the questions people have about my career to set the record straight as I seek to pass along the experience of my work.

The pharmacist's role as a provider is a current topic among many professional pharmacy organizations. In the United States, pharmacists are seen and depended upon, but they are often not valued by health care structures and, in some cases, even by other health care team members.

Yet, in many countries that I have been privileged to work in since 1980 – particularly those with developing economies – pharmacists have always been an unrecognized but dynamic provider of service in the communities in which they practice. They are often on the front line of health care. As I worked alongside them, one could see their practice move from solely the commercial to include the care continuum of health services.

I want young pharmacists to know that they have a set of skills that can be applicable in many, many settings. In the past, pharmacists were trained either to work in hospitals, community pharmacies, industrial settings, or academia. However, whenever medications are being discussed, pharmacists can have a seat at the table. They can contribute – whether it is in the context of policy, diplomacy, international health, or basic primary health care. But they have to show others at the table how those skills can be applied because other health professionals and policy makers may not yet understand.

Although it is changing, I have noticed that over the years, many in my profession have been minimally engaged with public health as a discipline. At the same time, many of those in public health are just now beginning to appreciate the role of the pharmacist. However, pharmacy and public health are both integral parts of the health care team. To be effective in producing good health outcomes in patients, you need to have both understandings. This chronicle is intended to shed some light on how we can do this for the betterment of every patient.

CHAPTER ONE

Embracing a Life of Service

For many people, a stellar career is one in which they excel in their profession or attain financial success and gain many awards or accolades. I define career success differently. I have always viewed my career as an opportunity to use the gifts God gave me and as a chance to serve God by serving my fellow man. Service, especially in the healing arts, is what has mattered the most to me. As George Washington Carver said, *"It is simply service that measures success."*

My initial interest in the healing arts was sparked by a bad case of eczema. As a child growing up in Harlem, I would experience breakouts so bad that I would miss days from school because of it. I remember having to take allergy shots and limit my diet because I was having such bad reactions to different foods. For a while, I could consume nothing but cottage cheese, tomatoes, goat milk, and pumpernickel bread.

While the experience was not pleasant, it was a turning point in my life. It was during this time that I was treated by two Black female physicians who practiced in Harlem – Hilda G. Straker and Daphne McCaskell. Not only did they treat my eczema, but they left me with an appreciation for the healing arts. I decided that I would pursue a career in medicine.

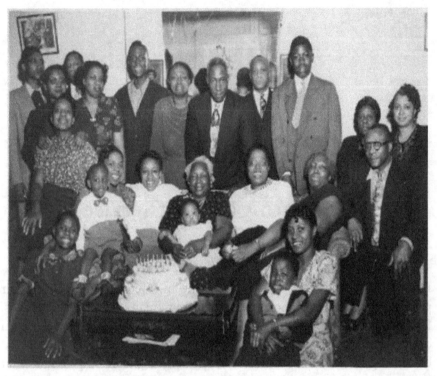

Family celebrating the 75th birthday of my great-grandmother, Nancy T. Handy. I am on front row left. (Courtesy of the author)

I was also inspired by family. My relatives always encouraged me to stretch myself and see past limitations – a skill that would serve me well throughout my career in pharmacy. When I was a child, my great-grandmother Nancy Handy, an orphan herself in Savannah, Georgia, would have me sit beside her and read the *New York Times* to her every day even though I didn't officially know how to read! She would tell me to sound the letters out, and I realized that when I applied myself, I could do more than I thought.

My mother, Ethel Jackson Cain Davis, taught me that work can be something of an adventure. My mother, who left Savannah at the age of 13, was one of the first high school graduates in the family, and she went on to work as a key punch operator at the War Department's Office of Dependency Benefits during World War II when the words 'data processing' were not in the common vernacular. As she wasn't in

20

a profession that many people knew about, such as a nurse or a doctor, members of my family would look at her and ask, "What are you doing again?" When I look back, I realize that she was running computers and IBM machines as she worked in various capacities within the Federal government long before most people even knew what IBM was! Today, one could say she certainly was one of the hidden figures in data processing.

By the time she retired, my mother was chief of the data processing branch of the Eastern Region for the Federal Aviation Agency. The fact that she achieved this level of authority with just a high school education showed me what is possible when you are persistent and stay true to a goal, no matter what. I have always drawn a lot of inspiration from her experiences and accomplishments, even when I was just discovering which professional path I would eventually take.

My father, Russell Samuel Cain, was a native of British Honduras and came to the U.S. on a ship, then stayed. He and my mother met at my Aunt Sue's café in Harlem and were married in 1937. They separated after I was born and she later married Floyd Davis, who raised me. From this new union I was blessed with a brother, Floyd Anthony Davis. Both men were hard-working: my father a tailor and businessman, and my step-father a WWII veteran and U.S. postal service employee.

Later in life, I would decide that pharmacy would be my career path of choice. However, early on I realized that pharmacists were largely underutilized in the healthcare system. We could do much more than stand behind the counter dispensing medication. There were many other opportunities for pharmacists to enhance patient care. As I worked as a pharmacist at Watts Health Clinic of Los Angeles, my eyes were opened and my vision was broadened about what I could do as a pharmacist, and how pharmacists could make a difference in the health care system as a whole, but especially for those who are underserved.

A Pioneering View of Pharmacy

My mother's career path had a profound impact on my life and taught me to dream big. The fact that my mother forged a way in a profession that was unheard of at the time taught me to look past the limitations of my own profession. The world looked at pharmacists one way, while I saw possibilities that many in the healthcare industry did not yet see.

After being the only pharmacist in my Master of Public Health program at the University of California Los Angeles in 1972, I knew that my purpose was somewhere at the intersection of pharmacy and public health. I began to focus on finding ways for pharmacists to serve and use their expertise within the healthcare team for the benefit of underserved patients. My activities began to shift from those of a traditional pharmacist to those of a pharmacist in public health – a role that was unheard of at that time.

I have always believed that pharmacists need to position themselves as frontline healthcare providers. But the medical world did not always see it that way. In the past, it was not customary for pharmacists to be consulted on matters of public health. Most people just looked at pharmacists as commercial beings, only there to dispense pills to patients. We weren't viewed as professionals with health training who could provide information; we were often seen merely as sellers of products. In fact, in the late 1960s, pharmacists were prohibited from discussing certain aspects of medication use with their patients.

However, I've always looked at things differently. Pharmacists were among the most accessible healthcare professionals, so it made sense to involve them in public health decisions. You don't need an appointment to see and speak to a pharmacist. There is no charge to speak to or secure advice from a pharmacist, and the wealth of knowledge that a pharmacist possesses is invaluable to patients' health.

I shared many of those views in an article I wrote along with Joel Kahn, B.S. Pharm in 1971 titled, "The Pharmacist as a Member of the Health Team." The article was published in the American Journal of Public Health in November of that same year. In the article, we described the changing role of the physician. We wrote:

The day of the physician acting in splendid isolation is also coming to an end. Paramedical personnel now with the team and increasing knowledge and skills upon which the physician must depend are shifting their perspective of the physician. They now view the physician as the coordinator of their efforts, and the channel through which their services affect total patient care.

About pharmacists, we wrote:

A pharmacist receives two to three times more training in pharmacology and drug therapeutics in pharmacy school than a physician does in medical school. The pharmacist of today has an up-to-date knowledge of drugs, including their therapeutic effect, posology, chemical composition, side effects, and contraindications. Students graduating from today's schools of pharmacy have also been educated in the recognition of drug interactions and in the enormous potential for their role in the prevention of iatrogenic diseases.... With this vast reservoir of scientific expertise at hand, why is the pharmacist called upon so infrequently to utilize and apply this information as it pertains to patient care?

That article was referenced in the American Society of Health-System Pharmacists (ASHP) Statement on the Role of Health-System Pharmacists in Public Health (1981) and even noted by such officials as James H. Cavanaugh, who served under President Richard Nixon as Staff Assistant to the President for Health Affairs, and Vernon E. Wilson, M.D., an Administrator with the Department of Health, Education, and Welfare. Wilson even wrote:

I am in general agreement with the main thrust of the article that the future of the pharmacist is as a member of a coordinated group of health professionals and para-

professionals.... The pharmacist's contribution to health care is a unique one. Whether it be through consultation with patients or prescribers, through participation in pharmacy and therapeutics committees, through the dissemination of drug-related health education material, through active monitoring of the drug habits of the patient, through the keeping of medication records, or through participation in drug abuse programs, the pharmacist makes a singular contribution to the coordinated delivery of health care.

A Passion for Serving the Underserved

I have particularly been driven to address pharmacy and public health needs in underserved communities. Perhaps that is because I was raised in Harlem, mostly in the Lincoln Projects in what would be described as an "underserved" or "underprivileged" community. While the people in my community may not have had a lot of money, I never felt like I was lacking anything.

The neighborhood was like a family, in that everybody knew one another, and everyone looked out for each other. In fact, through my upbringing, I learned first-hand what was meant by the concept, *'it takes a village.'* Looking out for others in the community has been a priority I have carried throughout my life.

Another reason I've embraced the idea of working with underserved communities is because I've witnessed the harm caused by stereotypes many people have about Black Americans, such as that we are disadvantaged underachievers and come from broken families. I wanted to right those misconceptions.

This passion stayed with me throughout my career – from the Watts Health Center, to the American Pharmaceutical (now Pharmacists) Association, to the United States Agency of International Development (USAID). It inspired me as I worked in twenty-two countries around the world and led the production of the first *Pharmaceuticals in Health*

Assistance program guidance for USAID. It influenced my thinking when I directed global health projects for Charles R Drew University of Medicine and Science, and later spearheaded the Office of International Programs (OIP) and the Pharmacists and Continuing Education (PACE) Center (a unique program that expanded the traditional practice skills of pharmacists in emerging or developing communities abroad) for Howard University School of Continuing Education.

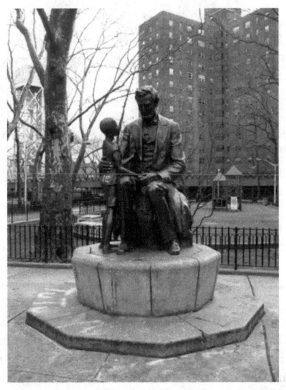

Picture of the project building in the Lincoln Projects near 135th Street and Park Avenue in Harlem. (https://jubiloemancipationcentury.wordpress.com/2015/07/07/ monument-lincoln-and-child-harlem-new-york/, accessed September 1, 2020)

Being a pharmacist with training in public health has given me an opportunity to realize my purpose in serving underserved communities around the world. It has also allowed me to push past limitations and help others to see that pharmacists could play an invaluable role in the healthcare system. But the road was not always easy.

CHAPTER TWO

Preparing for a Career in Pharmacy

Education has always been important to me. My family instilled in me the significance of doing well in school, and that served me well throughout my career. Every degree and training opportunity left me more prepared for the next.

I graduated from eighth grade at Harlem's All Saints Grammar School in 1951. Then in high school I was taught by the Sisters of Charity of NY for two years when I attended Cathedral High School - All Saints Branch, which was a premiere Catholic High School in New York City.

Around this time, my immediate family left the projects and moved to Hempstead, New York. My stepfather had recently come back from the war and he found work in the post office because it was an institution that was hiring Black men at the time. My family managed to purchase a little piece of property, a house out in Hempstead. Since this was about an hour and a half drive from Harlem, I left Cathedral High School to attend Hempstead High School and graduated from there in 1955.

Because of the excellent training I had received at Cathedral High School, I was put in advanced placement courses and ultimately graduated with honors. After that, I was offered scholarship assistance to attend Seton Hill College, a Catholic women's college in Greensburg, Pennsylvania run by the Sisters of Charity of Seton Hill. Today, the school is called

Seton Hill University, and it is a liberal arts university with approximately 2,500 students. To help me pay for schooling, I received the Cardinal Cushing Scholarship for Negroes, through the United Negro College Fund; I also received the Catholic Scholarship and Service for Negro Students.

My family also pitched in for me to go to school. Everybody helped out. My aunt was a seamstress and she made all my clothes – I was dressed to the nines. If a family member couldn't get me something for school, then they gave me a little piece of change. I also contributed to my education by working in the kitchen of Seton Hill as a part of the dishwashing team after dinner and made 50 cents an hour.

A Surprising Path

As I settled into life at Seton Hill College, I started inquiring as to what the Sisters of Charity of Seton Hill were all about. They were one of the orders of nuns formed by Elizabeth Ann Seton, the first American-born Saint canonized by the Roman Catholic Church in 1975. Their motto is *The Charity of Christ Urges Us,* and they were focused on service to the underserved. The more I learned about them, the more I liked what I saw. The idea of dedicating one's life to Christ drew me. At the end of my second year, I decided to become a postulant; I would take the first step in my calling to serve others as a nun.

While this decision may be surprising to those who hear about it today, my family has always been very, very spiritual. My great-grandmother was one of the founding members of Southern Baptist Church in Harlem. I've always known that I should put my trust in God and Jesus Christ. At Seton Hill, that message was reaffirmed for me, and again, my passion for serving the underserved was shared by everyone in the convent.

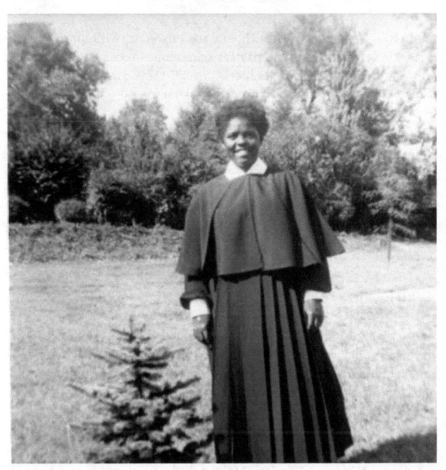

Rosalyn Maria Cain, Postulant, Sister of Charity of Seton Hill, Greensburg, PA, 1957
(Courtesy of the author)

The first stage of preparation to become a nun is called the Postulancy. During that time, I taught second grade at St. Bruno's Elementary School in Greensburg, Pennsylvania. On a typical day, I would get up at maybe 5:30 a.m. and go to chapel. I'd have my individual prayer, then participate in group prayer, then mass and finally breakfast, all before 8 a.m. Then I would go to work for the day teaching second graders at St. Bruno School in Greensburg, PA.

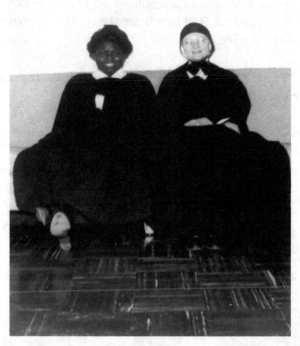

Postulant Rosalyn Maria Cain with Sister Harold Ann, Principal of St. Bruno's School (Courtesy of the author)

The next step in becoming a full-fledged nun was the Novitiate. During that year, I had no contact with the outside world. I could write letters to my family; they could write to me, but I could not go outside of the convent except for medical care purposes. It was a cloistered year of learning spiritual disciplines for being a nun. For example, I discovered that the discipline and routine of prayer on a regular basis allowed spiritual blessings to flow. That was also a time for me to discover more of what God wanted me to do. I became even more certain that I was called to serve. My relationship with God deepened, and I was more able to give greater recognition to the blessings that flowed.

At the end of the Novitiate, the Sisters of Charity knew that I had begun my studies at Seton Hill College with a major in chemistry and a minor in biology in preparation for medical school. They offered me an opportunity to go to pharmacy school, and I accepted. The Sisters of Charity had a convent in Pittsburgh at the Roselia Foundling & Maternity Home, and while living there, I could go to pharmacy school at Duquesne University.

I started pharmacy school in 1959, where I was the only African American studying pharmacy in my class. While there, I was elected to the Academic Honor Society in Pharmacy, Rho Chi Society, Alpha Beta chapter. I also interned at Pittsburgh Hospital, which at that time was run by the Sisters of Charity of Seton Hill. I received a Bachelor of Science in Pharmacy in 1962 as Sister Marie Martin, Sister of Charity.

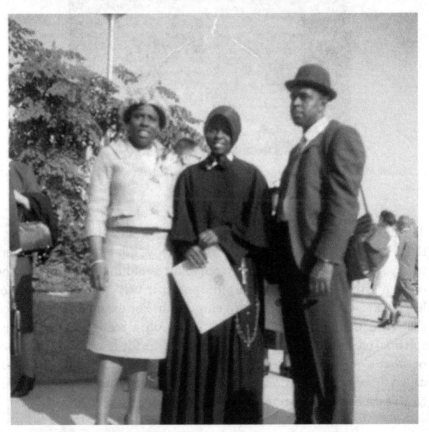

My mother, me, and my stepfather at graduation from Duquesne University, 1962 (Courtesy of the author)

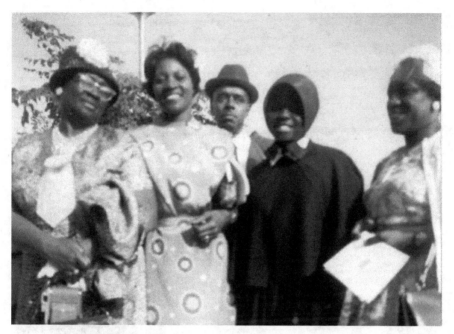

My grandmother Viola DuPrey, my aunt Dorothy Jackson, my stepfather Floyd Davis, me, and my aunt Emily Lawrence at my graduation from Duquesne University, 1962. (Courtesy of the author)

Being a pharmacist helped me to fulfill my purpose of pursuing a life of service. Pharmacists were well known in most communities and generally respected. They also played an important role in helping people to get their health needs met.

As a pharmacist-in-training at Pittsburgh Hospital, one had to work under a pharmacist; one could not work independently. However, the order wanted me to run the pharmacy at Pittsburgh Hospital by myself on the weekends. I didn't want to do that because doing so would jeopardize my licensing and path to pharmacy. This dilemma helped me to realize just how important a career in pharmacy was to me. The order and I could not come to terms, so in August 1962, I left the order and returned to Hempstead shortly after graduation.

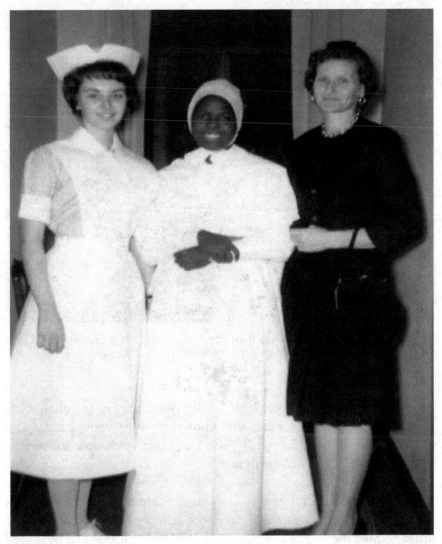

Sister Marie Martin, Servant of Charity, in uniform at Pittsburgh Hospital with student nurse and her mother. (Courtesy of the author)

Embracing a New Path

When I got back to Hempstead, I enrolled in St. John's University School of Pharmacy to pursue a Master of Science in Pharmacy, and was offered the opportunity to become a teaching assistant while working at a community pharmacy called Mardel's Pharmacy and Surgical Supply in Hempstead, NY. I did not complete my coursework at St. John's but later earned a Master's in Public Health from the University of California, Los Angeles (UCLA) in 1972. I earned this graduate-level degree because it was considered a key professional credential for working in public health.

At UCLA, I was the only pharmacist in my class. Many of my classmates wondered aloud why I was there and asked what role a pharmacist had in public health. When people would ask, I would point them to the *American Journal of Public Health* article that I wrote along with Joel Kahn, *"The Pharmacist as a Member of the Health Team."* I learned how to articulate what a pharmacist did and did not do within the sphere of health care at that time. It became important to speak not only to pharmacists but other health care professionals as well.

I earned a Doctor of Pharmacy from the University of Southern California (USC) in 1976. When I started pursuing my doctoral degree, I realized I had to be as prepared as possible to push back against people's perceptions about what pharmacists could and could not, and should and should not, do. I knew that furthering my education yet again would help me to bridge the worlds of pharmacy and public health even more.

While my early path to pharmacy and the education and training I received took many different turns, one thing remained constant throughout the entire journey – my commitment to serve. The convent helped me to develop the discipline that I needed to stay true to my purpose of serving those in need. The time I spent as a nun was also one of the many instances in my life where I was willing to go against the grain. Both of these attributes would serve me well as my career progressed.

CHAPTER THREE

Life as a Pharmacist in New York

When I returned to Hempstead after working at Pittsburgh Hospital, I knew I wanted to continue my work in pharmacy. It was 1962, which was long before the days of chain drug stores like CVS. At that time Mardel's Pharmacy and Surgical Supply was considered one of the major pharmacies in Hempstead, NY– as its location indicated. It was right across from Abraham & Straus, which was the big department store (like today's Dillard's or Macy's) on the city's main thoroughfare. The pharmacy was on the street level. Upstairs, there was a laboratory, as well as a fitting room for surgical garments, and an area where surgical supplies were sold.

One day, I went into the pharmacy and asked if they were hiring; they interviewed me, and I was hired at a pay rate of $1.25 per hour for a 40-hour work week though I had no benefits at the time. I believe that my background working in the pharmacy at Pittsburgh Hospital played a big role in my being hired for that job.

I learned a lot at Mardel's. I compounded and dispensed prescriptions, and I purchased surgical and cosmetic supplies. I also completed a course on the fitting of surgical and orthopedic garments, after which I received an S.H. CAMP (Samuel Higby Camp) certificate.

It was also there that I learned about the value of authenticity in the workplace and how important it is to share your true self. I remember one experience in particular. During my time at Mardel's, I was the only woman and African American pharmacist on staff. I wanted to travel to Washington, D.C. to take part in the March on Washington in August of 1963. I was told that I risked losing my job if I decided to go, but I went anyway. When I came back, I was surprised when the owner and all the other pharmacists asked me plenty of questions about the experience. They wanted to know my impressions of the march. I shared what insights I could, and there was no word of a firing!

From Community Pharmacy Back to the Hospital

After working at Mardel's for two years, I moved to New York City in 1964. For a summer, I worked at Harlem Hospital where I'd been born. I then took a job as a staff pharmacist at Lenox Hill Hospital in 1965. I was excited to be a part of what was then well-regarded as an innovative hospital pharmacy; its director at that time, Gilbert Simon, was known nationally. Back then, Lenox Hill was just starting a new process called the "unit dose" system. Through this system, once a medication left the pharmacy, it was charged to a patient, whether it was used or not. Unused, prepackaged tablets and capsules could be returned to the pharmacy for a patient credit. Our pharmacy also prepared and sterilized basic I.V. solutions.

I worked in the inpatient and outpatient sections of the pharmacy, filling prescriptions, getting pharmaceuticals ready for later use, and ensuring the sterile packaging of ophthalmic preparations. I was also involved in the general professional supervision of technical staff.

One of the biggest challenges I faced in this role was balancing communication with the nursing team and physicians. At Lenox Hill Hospital, as at other medical facilities of the time, physicians prescribed, pharmacists dispensed, and nurses administered the medications. Pharmacists were not yet regarded as the medication experts they are. But when the nurses had questions or concerns about the medications that physicians prescribed, they would go to the pharmacists, not the doctors. Mediating relationships between the professions was tough at times.

I also had to get used to the location of the pharmacy, which was in the basement of the hospital where there was little or no contact with the rest of the hospital or the patients. This was a challenge for me, especially having come from Pittsburgh Hospital, where the pharmacy was on the main floor of a highly trafficked hall. Its location allowed pharmacists to easily build a good camaraderie with the nurses and nursing supervisors who were fellow nuns. That wasn't the case at Lenox Hill Hospital.

To help improve and strengthen communication between pharmacists, nurses, and physicians at Lenox Hill, I frequently went to the floor to check "floor stock" quantities and expiration dates of medications while monitoring scheduled drug administrations. Doing so gave me and the other pharmacists better access to the two professions as they practiced and improved the dynamics of the patient care process.

My time at Lenox Hill planted the seeds for the work I would do in the future to advocate for expanding the pharmacist's role. There was so much that my fellow pharmacists and I could offer beyond being pill-counters. I was convinced that the health care system would be so much more effective and that patients would be better served if the skills and talents of pharmacists were better utilized.

I've learned in my life and career that you never know how others will impact you. A conversation can spark a new idea that takes your life in an entirely different direction. That's what happened to me after a few years of working at Lenox Hill Hospital.

When I worked at Mardel's, there was a fellow pharmacist named Isaac (Ike) Behar. He left Mardel's and moved to Los Angeles with his wife and two daughters. Years later, after talking to some former colleagues from Mardel's, I found out that Ike was making $6.25 an hour as a pharmacist in California after making $1.25 an hour at Mardel's. When I learned about the money he was earning, I considered what it would be like to move to California for the first time. I was young and adventurous and decided that California was worth exploring. As life would have it, my career took another major turn. I left Lenox Hill and headed west.

CHAPTER FOUR

The Move to Los Angeles

When I arrived in California, I faced one immediate obstacle: my pharmacist license was for New York, not California. But there was a Veterans Affairs clinic out there, and with the federal government, if pharmacists are duly licensed in one state, they can work within the system. So, I worked at the Veterans Affairs clinic for a few months until I got my California license. Working there taught me that I did not want to work at a mail order pharmacy. I enjoyed working with, educating, and helping patients one-on-one. But at the clinic, I had very little or no contact with patients. Because there was such little interaction, I couldn't get a good feel for what patients needed regarding their medicines.

Once I was licensed, I got a job as pharmacist in charge at Thrifty Drugs, a major drug store chain in Los Angeles. I dispensed and compounded prescriptions and provided drug information to prescribers and patients.

While at Thrifty Drugs, I rotated through several stores, including one store downtown on 6th Street and another at Rodeo Road and La Brea Avenue. The store on Rodeo and La Brea was one of their busiest – it wasn't unheard of for me to fill 150 prescriptions during my eight-hour shift! I was so busy that I had little time to talk to customers. I often had to call on the store clerk to assist in ringing up the prescription sales. Consultations on prescriptions were at the bare minimum.

There was a pause in my work as a pharmacist with Thrifty Drugs as I found myself expecting my daughter. During this period, I stopped working as a pharmacist and became a nanny until I delivered, after which I went back to Thrifty. God provides; the wife of one of my colleagues at Thrifty Drugs cared for children. She helped care for my daughter, allowing me to move forward in my career, and later, my education.

An Expanded Role for Pharmacists

During his State of the Union address in 1964, President Lyndon B. Johnson introduced legislation known as the War on Poverty. One of the initiatives that came under it was the establishment of neighborhood health centers in medically underserved inner city and rural areas of the country, first at Tufts University in 1965, and Mound Bayou in Mississippi that same year. These health centers, established by the Office of Economic Opportunity (OEO), aimed to provide disenfranchised populations access points to health and social services. Initially called "neighborhood health centers" as a War on Poverty demonstration program, they were intended to serve as a mechanism for community empowerment. (*Sardell, The U.S. Experiment in Social Medicine: The Community Health Center Progam 1965-1986, University of Pittsburgh Press, 1988*). The health centers were designed and run with extensive community involvement to ensure that they remained responsive to the community's needs.

One of the first eight established was the South Central Multipurpose Health Services Center in Watts, Los Angeles. It later became the Watts Health Center, and is now the Watts Health Foundation. Initially, it was under the leadership of the University of Southern California (USC), but in 1969 the grant was transferred from USC to the Community Board.

I first learned about the Watts Health Center while watching television in 1967. There was a story about the Center's groundbreaking that captured my interest. I called and asked if they needed a pharmacist. When they said yes, I applied and got the job of senior pharmacist to serve with Garner V. Grayson, a well-known black pharmacist in Los Angeles, and the center's Chief Pharmacist.

When I compared New York to Watts, I initially thought Watts was paradise. Unlike New York, Watts had trees, and there were houses with driveways and garages. However, upon a closer look, I noticed that there were no stores, play areas, or theaters. In fact, the Watts neighborhood seemed cut off, and it lacked many of the services that other neighborhoods received from Los Angeles County. This is where I needed to be.

Watts is where I began to spread my wings as a pharmacist. In addition to dispensing and procuring drugs, Mr. Grayson gave me the job of developing an operational model for the pharmacy. The center formally developed a health care team composed of clinicians including physicians, dentists, nurses, social workers, and neighborhood health agents, and I was asked to lead the team in the development of ways to use pharmacists' skills and knowledge innovatively.

One of my innovative techniques was to teach pharmacology updates to a class of nurses. I also edited and published a monthly pharmacy in-service sheet titled "Capsules." In addition, I trained and supervised two pharmacists, two technicians, and one clerk. With such a wide range of duties, I had the opportunity to use all my training as a pharmacist. I was grateful for the pharmacist director, Mr. Grayson, who had vision and allowed my ideas to flow.

My time at Watts also made me realize the tremendous influence the pharmacy's placement in the facility had on patient interaction. At Watts Health Center, the pharmacy was near the front door in the front lobby. We were the last health professionals to see patients at the end of their encounters within the facility, so our pharmacists could cement or reinforce important instructions and recommendations the patient had received about their medications.

Watts Health Center used the concept of the neighborhood health agent. Neighborhood health agents were people from the community who were trained to go into homes and serve as a connection between the residents and the health center. They could help people make appointments and learn how the health center could be of service.

At this time, I instituted the practice of pharmacists going with the neighborhood health agents during their visits, and with permission, actually looking inside of residents' medicine cabinets. The pharmacists would then talk with residents about their medications and any problems or adverse effects they were experiencing. We found that many people were not taking their medications properly, and some didn't even know the difference between several medications they were taking.

In some cases, people were taking different medications for a variety of ailments and those medications sometimes interacted. During these visits, our pharmacists made presentations on the proper use of medicines. I even had a saying that I used to repeat: "There's not a pill for every ill." Many people think they can go to the pharmacy for any ailment, but I would remind them that each of us only has one body, so we might not be able to take a pill for everything. And, most of all, all the pills being taken were for the same body!

By speaking with residents face-to-face, pharmacists were able to contribute to their healthier living. This was a clear example of pharmacists making a difference in the world of public health. Going out and speaking to members of the community removed me from "mind-mechanizing" tasks such as counting and pouring, and directed me to "mind-blowing" activities, such as being part of a vibrant, innovative health care team. Under my leadership at the Watts Health Center, pharmacists began to formally serve as a drug information resource, as a drug monitoring and management colleague, and as developers of procedures for home evaluation of patients' medicine use, among other things.

I was the youngest pharmacist out of the professional staff of four. Because of my age, I often felt that I had to prove myself. In other words, I had to "put up or shut up." However, my ideas were respected and typically used by the director.

The chief of pharmacy, Garner V. Grayson Jr., later wrote a letter of recommendation that described the impact my work had on the organization. In part, he wrote:

During Miss Cain's employment here at the Center, I became more and more aware of her keen insight into the community needs, as well as her fine ability as a professional pharmacist. She became involved in several constructive programs, taught Pharmacology to a class of nurses, edited and published a monthly pharmacy in-service sheet called "Capsules," and was a guiding influence in our Center Professional Organization.

Because of Miss Cain's previous hospital experience back East, her knowledge was extremely valuable to me in setting up pharmacy procedures here in the Center. She maintained a fine professional relationship with the physicians and dentists in the Center and was often called upon to assist them in various programs.

I was energized by this work, and I could clearly see the difference between having a *job* and having a *calling*. I also began to expand my notion of what a pharmacist could do. A person with my training and background had a lot to offer, not only to those who get their prescriptions filled but to my colleagues in the pharmacy profession. Little did I know that I would play a role in helping to shape people's perceptions of what a pharmacist could do.

CHAPTER FIVE

A Different Direction

My work at the Watts Health Center, prepared me for the next big step in my career. In 1969, the American Pharmaceutical Association (APhA), now called the American Pharmacists Association, recruited me to be the assistant director of a research project funded by the Office of Economic Opportunity (OEO). We would study ways to improve services to impoverished communities served by community health centers. The project was called, "The Delivery of Pharmaceutical Services to Poverty Areas of the United States."

I was recommended for the position by Mary Louise Andersen, a pharmacy leader who later became the first female Speaker of the House of Delegates for the American Pharmacists Association. She was intrigued by the work we were doing in Watts. She was visiting Los Angeles and decided to stop by the health center. The two of us hit it off, and I remember that we went to dinner and ended up talking until two or three in the morning. I explained to her all of the innovative ways that our pharmacists were providing services to the local community. I also shared with her the model we developed at Watts, which was later published in the *American Journal of Pharmaceutical Education, Volume 14, December 1970.*

The model components included, among others, and in addition to the traditional drug distribution function, the following fifteen items:

1. Consultation with patients on prescription medication and related items
2. Consultation with health center prescribers in the choice of a drug
3. Participation in a Pharmacy and Therapeutics Committee
4. Active participation on a family health team with health agents
5. Health education
6. In-service education
7. Manpower development
8. Medication follow-up for renewal
9. Taking medication histories
10. Acting in a patient advocate role
11. Coordination of drug therapy
12. Establishing Drug Abuse Control policies
13. Going into a patient's home with health agents to assure patient compliance with the medication regimen in the home
14. Teaming with an RN to handle health screening, health maintenance and primary medical care
15. Assigning a pharmacist to a center's unit to do health screening and drug monitoring; and assigning a pharmacist to a medical unit to handle all prescription decisions upon the presentation of diagnosis and/or symptoms by the physician

The elements in this model served as a springboard for models still being used today.

When Mary Louise Andersen returned to Washington, D.C., she reported back to William S. Apple, the executive director of the APhA at the time. She recommended that I be a part of the project because I had so much experience working with the community health center in Watts. I had no idea that she was going to recommend me. In fact, I had no idea that they were getting ready to do this project at all.

The announcement of my new role in the APhA newsletter on August 23, 1969, described my professional experiences that were crucial to me being offered the position:

Miss Cain, who has a background in community and hospital pharmacy, has been serving as Senior Staff Pharmacist at the South Central Multipurpose Health Services Center in Los Angeles. In addition to her duties as a pharmacist in this position, Miss Cain served as In-Service Coordinator, In-Service Instructor to the Nursing Department, Editor of the In-Service Pharmacy Bulletin and Assistant to the Chief Pharmacist in the organization, development and innovation of the pharmacy system of the health center.

Miss Cain's community pharmacy experience was gained in Los Angeles and Hempstead, New York, and her hospital pharmacy experience in Brooklyn Hospital and Lenox Hospital, New York, and Pittsburgh Hospital, Pennsylvania.... She is a member of the APhA, American Society of Hospital Pharmacists and Rho Chi.

Working for the national professional association of pharmacists had a special appeal to me. I did not know when I got there that I was going to be the first African American professional pharmacist on staff. That, in itself, was exciting. I also developed a new appreciation for the history of pharmacists in the United States, though at the time, that history did not include many of the contributions of Black and other minority pharmacists. That fact inspired a later article co-authored in American Druggist with Dr. Ira C. Robinson in 1978 titled, *"Black Pharmacists in the U.S. and How Their Status is Changing."*

The job with the APhA required a move from Los Angeles to Washington, D.C. The APhA headquarters was on the corner of 23rd Street and Constitution Avenue, and it is still in that location today. In fact, it was and is the only privately owned plot of land on Constitution Avenue, which faces the National Mall. (https://www.washingtonpost. com/lifestyle/style/the-curious-story-of-the-malls-lone-privately-owned-plot/2017/10/18/9d894632-b27e-11e7-9e58-e6288544af98_story.html, accessed 2/5/ 2020) In 2009, the Association added a second annex to the building and now the State Department leases some of the space. The initial front section of the building, the historic part, remains. That was the location of my office. I had the distinct privilege to work in the historic sections of both APhA and the U.S. State Department across the street. More on that later.

Several years ago, as a fundraising effort, APhA allowed the purchase of engraved bricks, or pavers, on the East Terrace of the building. I bought one and had it placed under the window where I used to work. So, my name is on Constitution Avenue engraved in stone! The paver reads: *Rosalyn C. King, PharmD, MPH, RPh, Ass't Proj Dir, APhA/OEO Proj, 1969-1971.*

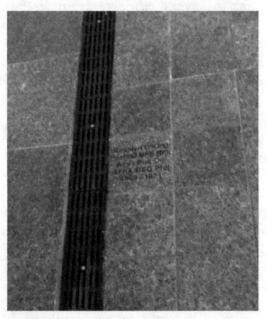

The paver on the East Terrace of the American Pharmacist Association/State Department building with my name on it. (Courtesy of the author)

When I got to Washington, D.C., one of the first orders of business was to find housing. I went to the Pentagon Housing Office to look at their list of available apartments in the area. When I chose one near the Navy Annex, the resident manager told me that no apartments were available, even though I knew that was untrue. I told the APhA executive director, William S. Apple, and he sent his secretary out to try and rent the apartment; she found that the apartment was, indeed, available.

I went to the local American Civil Liberties Union (ACLU) office and they sent a letter to the landlord indicating that the Pentagon would be informed that they were discriminating against potential tenants. Soon after, the landlord called me and told me the apartment was available but would not be ready for a month. The office of the executive director of the APhA had an apartment for short-term use by visitors, and he made it available for me until I could move into my apartment. It was a penthouse overlooking the Potomac. I was always moved by the fact that he did not hesitate to assist in my search for housing.

Settling in at the APhA

My new role at APhA was different from anything I had done in the past. I no longer filled prescriptions; the project was fully focused on policy and programs. I also had no contact with patients other than when I went on site visits to health centers around the country.

There were three pharmacists on the team: Pharmacist Sydney P. Galloway was director of the project, and Joel S. Kahn and I were the assistant project directors. We weren't your traditional working group. There was one man of Jewish ancestry, one man considered a WASP (White Anglo-Saxon Protestant), and me. In fact, there was a television program on at that time called the Mod Squad about three outsiders – a white man, a black man, and a woman – who worked together to solve crimes. Our team was given that nickname by other members of the APhA staff. They would have official board meetings and they would ask the Mod Squad to come and attend.

As I was the first African American on the Association staff, it's not too surprising that there were cultural differences that I and others had to work through. For example, one of my favorite letter closings at the time was "Keep on Keepin' On." The secretary had never heard the expression, and if asked to type it, would repeat it, except she would always add a 'g' to the end of 'keepin'." I had to explain to her that the 'g' wasn't part of the saying. I preferred the colloquial saying to the usual Standard English grammar.

Experiences like that gave me a new appreciation for my background growing up in Harlem of the 40's and 50's. Living in New York, I had the opportunity to interact with persons of differing cultures, languages, and faiths. That helped me to work with people of all backgrounds in this position.

One of the first steps in the project was to conduct a comprehensive survey of medical, pharmaceutical, and social literature to discover what research already existed on the delivery of pharmaceutical services in poverty areas. There wasn't much. In "Pharmacy in Poverty Areas – A Literature Search," our team wrote:

> *The small volume of relevant information retrieved from this literature review is indicative of the lack of research completed in this particular area of pharmacy practice. The need for such information complements the current trends in pharmaceutical practice and education; that is, a shifting of emphasis from drugs and drug products toward the physiological and social needs of the patient.*

The project centered on us making contact with neighborhood health centers around the country and deciding whether or not to include their experiences in the research. If we did, we had to determine how to categorize their experience. The work entailed talking with pharmacists attending various regional conferences to explain what it was we were doing. We spent a lot of time on the road conducting surveys, making presentations, and sharing results with the profession. The highlight for me was visiting the neighborhood health centers.

I also received a crash course in Washington politics. That's when I learned how the government really functioned at its various organizational levels. I could see very clearly what you had to do to keep your program going and which relationships you had to manage up and down that organizational chain. In fact, managing relationships took almost as much time as doing the work. That was a key insight for me, and it would help me later when I worked with the federal government.

As a matter of protocol, among the first things I did when I came to Washington was to visit the Howard University (HU) College of Pharmacy and meet with its Dean. Dr. Chauncey I. Cooper, the founding Dean of the School of Pharmacy at HU and the founder of the National Pharmaceutical Association (a professional association for minority pharmacists), was quite formidable. Besides being the only College of Pharmacy in Washington D.C., it was a Historically Black College/University (HBCU). Concurrently, APhA was seeking to have a greater involvement of minority pharmacists in all of its sections, including the Student American Pharmaceutical Association (SAPhA), and HU had a group of students interested in involvement with SAPhA.

In preparation for an upcoming SAPhA meeting in 1970, HU students expressed interest in becoming active with SAPhA. This was well received by APhA until it was recognized that the HU students wanted to be a part of the leadership of SAPhA. Sharon Roquemore (now Sharon L. Edwards) stepped forward to run as a vice-presidential candidate; Anthony Rogers ran for another office. By the time of the election, a good group of HU students had gotten geared up for involvement in SAPhA. However, both HU candidates lost and when the voting process was questioned, the APhA advisor did not entertain any suggestions regarding review of the process. At that point, the HU students and other minority students in attendance walked out of the meeting and abandoned any notion of active participation with the SAPhA.

It was after the election rebuff that discussion began on forming a student group and aligning with the National Pharmaceutical Association (NPhA). At the time, NPhA was not perceived to be as active within the profession as the students desired. However, with persuasion from myself, expressions from Texas Southern University's (TSU) Mickey Leland, and NPhA leadership, primarily Dean Cooper, the seed germinated.

In 1972, the Student National Pharmaceutical Association was officially founded on the campus of Florida Agriculture and Mechanical University (FAMU). Though not at the FAMU 1972 meeting as some have suggested, I was heavily involved in the decision and preparations to form a student group and align it with NPhA. Already a graduated and licensed pharmacist as well as an employee of APhA, I was precluded from being a founding student member, but was privileged to work with Sharon Roquemore, John Scrivens, Henry Lewis and others to offer mentorship, advice, and guidance during the time I worked at APhA and afterwards, when asked.

Early involvement with SNPhA was acknowledged in August, 1992, when the SNPhA Executive Director, Marisa Lewis, asked me to join in a commemorative program, "Walk Down Memory Lane," and share what I knew of the backstory that led up to the founding of SNPhA. She noted in her follow-up letter:

> *Please accept our gratitude for participating in the SNPhA 20th Annual National Convention. Thank you especially for participating in 'Walk Down Memory Lane.' We were all touched by reflections and by the history lesson. I feel this was the highlight of the meeting.*

Overall, my time at APhA solidified for me the role pharmacists could, should, and needed to play in the contribution to patient care. The landmark study that I worked on also expanded on the model I had used in Watts and articulated many of the ways that pharmacists in various health care organizations could increase their contributions to health services. Throughout the time of the study, the Deans of all four HBCU Schools of Pharmacy schools reached out to me with encouragement and requests for speaking engagements while I was at APhA. In addition to Howard University, those schools were Texas Southern in Houston, Texas; Xavier University in New Orleans, Louisiana; and Florida A&M in Tallahassee (FAMU), Florida.

When the project was over, I joined my colleagues as co-author of the final project report. The principles and constructs are still in use by many today when considering service to the underserved in poverty areas.

CHAPTER SIX

The Charles R Drew Postgraduate
Medical School Years

(In 1987, the School formally became the Charles R. Drew
University of Medicine and Science)

While working at APhA, I thought about going back to school to further my education. Our project director, Sydney Galloway, had a Master of Public Health. It was uncommon for a pharmacist to have that degree, but I wondered how the degree could help my service.

In 1970, one of the trips I had to take for APhA work was to Portland, Oregon. After I left Portland, I stopped in Los Angeles, my old stomping grounds, and decided to visit UCLA to explore the potential of going to its School of Public Health. As fate would have it, that's when I met the man who would become my husband, Sterling King Jr. He was in UCLA's student affairs office when I arrived there.

Near the end of my contract with APhA in 1971, I decided to move back to Los Angeles to enroll at UCLA. We were in the process of completing the report and the team agreed that we would continue co-authoring and commenting on the documents even though I was in Los Angeles. I remember that we sent documents back and forth overnight, all as I was getting myself in gear to go to school. Formally, in the fall of 1971, I became the only pharmacist in my Master of Public Health program.

My article had appeared in the *American Journal of Public Health,* and now was the time to fully educate myself on the rubrics of public health. My public health calling was building.

Impactful Days at Drew

During this time, the Charles R. Drew Postgraduate Medical School was still in its early formation stages. It was a growing institution and very clearly aligned with health services for the Watts, Willowbrook, and Compton areas. It was very clear that community medicine was the school's big thrust.

One day, I called Dr. Moses Alfred Haynes, who was then the chairman of the Department of Community and Preventive Medicine in the school, and discussed with him the possibility of working with Drew. I didn't know then that he was also a member of the faculty in the School of Public Health at UCLA.

He had a particularly strong interest in seeing that the Black and other minority students had opportunities such as internships. He offered me a role as a research analyst for one of the programs that he directed called the MEDEX Program.

In 1971 and early 1972, my job for the MEDEX Program was to be a part of the functional task analysis team. Functional task analysis is credited as leading to what is now often called task shifting. We were charged with trying to identify where MEDEXs could use the skills they acquired for the betterment of patient care. As part of our process, we analyzed the different tasks that physicians performed and investigated whether the skill level of a physician was required to perform them. If MEDEX could perform them, this would help meet the physician shortage of the time.

The MEDEXs were those persons who were trained in the military as independent medical duty corpsmen. The concept was introduced by Dr. Richard Smith in his physician-extender approach. MEDEXs were people who had been on the battlefield; they could do triage; they could do all kinds of assessments; some of them could even do surgery. But when they came home, there was no place for them within the healthcare sphere to use those skills. So, we were then charged with trying to identify where they could use those acquired skills to the betterment of patient care. We also looked at how MEDEXs compared to physician's assistants. There was a heavy similarity, except physician's assistants may not have had that battlefield experience.

Functional task analysis had a major impact on how a healthcare team could work. We would take the more highly skilled person and match them with a person with a lower level of training. In terms of time and cost, the strategy was advantageous because it optimized the role of each person. Those with a lower level of training can take on tasks they can competently perform while freeing the more specialized trained person to perform higher levels of care.

The MEDEX Project was tedious activity, but insightful and incredibly exciting. All these new concepts about how people work within the healthcare system and how they can use their skills in productive ways to influence outcome reinforced my views about the expanding role of pharmacists. The MEDEX Project also helped me to question how to contribute to a system of healthcare that is responsive to the needs of the community. Drew's focus on Community Medicine was another eye-opening exercise. We had to consider not only the population, but the environment, the levels of income, and all of the demographics of the community. We also had to strategize about how to deliver services to the community in a culturally competent manner.

Around 1972, Dr. Haynes was asked to develop an ambulatory evaluation team for the federal government. It was called the Drew Ambulatory Care Review Team (DART), and it was one of two teams that evaluated all government-funded community health center programs in the United States. The other was the Albert Einstein Medical College Team of New York's Albert Einstein University.

From the beginning to 1976, I had two jobs on the DART team: I was one of the site coordinators, which required that I administer all the logistics around each of the site visits; I also served as the pharmacy, lab, and x-ray services evaluator. Since we evaluated pharmaceutical services in more than three dozen community health centers across the United States, traveling was the norm. We were gone about twice a month.

Between May 1973 and October 1976, we conducted evaluations, and here is a sample of the health center sites visited:

• Northeast Valley Health Corporation in San Fernando Valley, California;
• Alviso Family Health Center in Alviso, California;
• Lee County Cooperative Clinic in Marianna, Arkansas;
• Miles Square Health Center in Chicago, Illinois;
• Medgar Evers Comprehensive Healthcare Center in Fayette, Mississippi;
• Wayne Miner Comprehensive Health Center in Detroit, Michigan;
• Pilot City Health Service Neighborhood Health Center in Minneapolis, Minnesota;
• Denver Neighborhood Health Program in Denver, Colorado;
• North East Medical Services in San Francisco, California;
• Jefferson Comprehensive Care Center in Pine Bluff, Arkansas;
• Atlanta Southside Comprehensive Health Center in Atlanta, Georgia;
• Mission Neighborhood Health Center in San Francisco, California;
• North County Health Project in San Marcus, California;
• Hough Norwood Neighborhood Health Center in Cleveland, Ohio;
• Medical Care Center of Louisiana, INC. in New Orleans, Louisiana;
• Ambulatory Services of Meharry Medical College-Matthew Walker Comprehensive Health Center in Nashville, Tennessee;
• Madison-Yazoo-Leake Family Health Center in Canton, Mississippi;

- Anchorage Neighborhood Health Center in Anchorage, Alaska;
- Mary Mahoney Memorial Health Center in Oklahoma City, Oklahoma;
- Waianae Coast Comprehensive Health Center in Waianae, Hawaii;
- Community Health Foundation of East Los Angeles, California;
- Centro de Salud Familiar La Fe in El Paso, Texas;
- Centro de Salud de La Comunidad de San Ysidro Community Health Center in San Diego, California; and
- Hunts Point Multiservice Center in Bronx, NY.

We created a project report on the evaluation of pharmaceutical services in community health centers from our work on the DART team. It was published in *Contemporary Pharmacy Practice* in 1979. Many of the concepts that we described in the report are forerunners of pharmacy practice evaluation today.

My experience at the DART and MEDEX programs taught me the importance of teamwork and community, and why an effective team had to be able to meld skills to achieve goals. I enjoyed working with a whole constellation of Black health professionals during my time at Drew. Dr. Haynes was a mentor to many Black public health professionals, including former Surgeon General David Satcher, and Dr. Richard Smith, developer of the MEDEX concept. They were inspirations for our team as they were always developing innovative ways of doing things – many of which are still done today. For example, David Satcher organized the very first health fair that I know of in a church – Second Baptist Church in Los Angeles – *in the early 1970s*. Today, it is not unusual to attend a health fair in a church. That's the kind of cauldron we were working in.

Throughout my career, I was always involved in professional associations. During this time, I became active in the National Pharmaceutical Foundation, which is now defunct. As part of the American Public Health Association, I served with many others in the structuring of its Black Caucus of Health Workers. For the work in APhA and Watts, I was awarded the Black Caucus of Health Workers of the American

Public Health Association's nationally prestigious Hildrus A. Poindexter Distinguished Service Award in 1976.

Second National Pharmaceutical Foundation Symposium, 1977

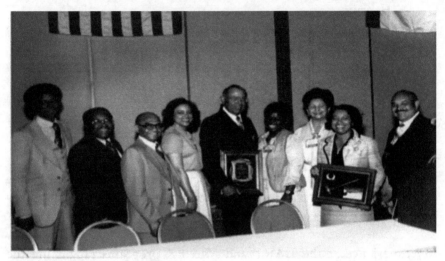

Left to right: Ted Matthews, Ira Robinson, Roy Darlington, Marie Best, Clyde Hatch, Rosalyn C. King, Ramona McCarthy, Mary Munson Runge, Pat Wells
(Courtesy of Dr. Ira C. Robinson)

Locally, my involvement was still strong with the Central Los Angeles Pharmaceutical Association (CLAPA), and in March, 1975, I was installed as President of the organization by Mary Munson Runge, who later became the first female and first African American President of the American Pharmacists Association in 1979.

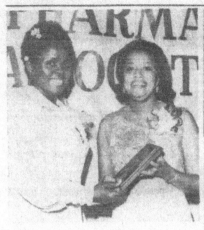

Thursday, March 20, 1975   Los Angele

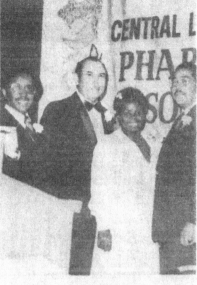

PLANS TO ASSIST Pharmaceutical students through scholarship and encouragement was evidenced during Installation Banquet of Central Los Angeles Pharmaceutical Association, recently. Presentation of award to Mrs. Mary Munson, state president of the association, is made by Rosalyn Cain King, left, newly installed president of CLAPA. Mrs. Munson, of Oakland, California has made outstanding contributions to the profession of pharmacy.

1975 OFFICERS, stand proudly beneath the Pharmaceutical Bo Marriott Hotel. From left, Joseph Almeida, director of Assoc Rosalyn Cain King, president; Gilbert Mathieu, vice preside Nadler, secretary.

CONVERSATION ON DAIS, probably focuses on future plans of new cabinet of CLAPA. The group was founded in 1966 to serve the needs of pharmacists in the Central L.A. region. From left, below, Clyde Hatch, Sterling King, Jr., Rosalyn Cain King

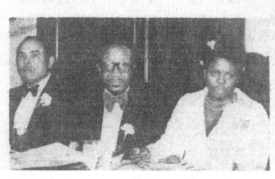

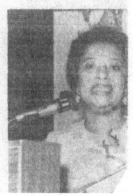

(Los Angeles Sentinel Newspaper, Courtesy of Los Angeles County Library, Black Resource Center)

Also, in 1976, I was nominated to the California State Board of Pharmacy. In a letter of recommendation sent to the Honorable Edmund G. Brown,

Jr, the governor of the state of California at the time, Congressman Julian Dixon, wrote:

> *Mrs. King is a pharmacist with a vast background not only in her profession, but in community-oriented health programs. She is highly respected in both her profession and community and has the education, experience, and desire to serve on this board. Her appointment would definitely be an asset to the people of California.*

My nomination, however, was not developed as I would eventually leave California that same year to accompany my husband to Howard University in Washington, D.C.

The insights I gained during this period of my career helped form my views about the role that pharmacists could play as an integral part of the health care team. During that time, I had the opportunity to expand my thinking, and I learned new approaches, strategies, and techniques that I would take with me throughout my career.

Between 1972 and 1976, everything I did in my career was at an organizational level; I was no longer involved in individual patient care, though I continued to get my pharmacy license renewed in case I ever needed to return to dispensing. At this point, my path took a clearer turn toward the broader aspects of public health.

CHAPTER SEVEN

A Crash Course in Business

I didn't know when I met Dr. M. Alfred Haynes and his wife, Hazel Edgecombe Haynes, how large of a role they would play in my professional life. In 1977, my career took another turn when my husband, Sterling, and I formed a business venture under the leadership of Dr. and Mrs. Haynes. I served as vice president of a company in Bethesda, Maryland called SECON Inc. Dr. Haynes was the president.

SECON was an acronym for Systems Evaluation of Care Consultants. What we had in mind to do was to improve and take into the commercial realm the Systems Evaluation of Care concept and process that had been developed by Dr. Haynes as he led various teams and consultancies.

Up until that time, the evaluation of healthcare was always talked about in terms of structure, process, and outcome. Dr. Haynes, however, was concerned with the concept of 'transformation of care.' What happens to the patient to transform them from a sick person to a well person? What does the system do within that transformation? The idea was to look at a patient when she or he first came in the door, and again when they were leaving, in order to discover what happened in that whole transformational process. That was significant.

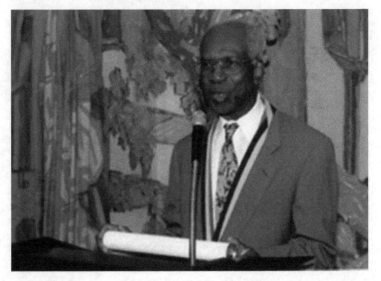

Dr. M. Alfred Haynes (Courtesy of the Haynes Family)

We took those concepts and worked with a lot of other teams in different healthcare centers to apply them so those healthcare centers could improve their services.

Here are some of the many highlight during my time at SECON, Inc:

- We conducted evaluations for the Department of Health Education and Welfare, Health Services Administration (DHEW/HSA).
- We produced evaluation manuals and tools that other healthcare organizations could use.
- We trained community health programs on methods of self-improvement.
- The United States Agency for International Development (USAID) awarded us a contract to provide technical assistance for their primary health care project evaluations.
- Howard University also hired us. The University asked us to come in and assess their College of Medicine for the potential of offering a program in public health. We did the assessment and created a report, and they took our recommendations.

Entrepreneurial Lessons

Though we were focused on improving healthcare, this was also the time that I learned about structuring and operating a business. I saw first-hand the importance of the structure and the function of a company. For example, I didn't know what a Subchapter S Corporation was until we had to form one. I had no idea about key man insurance until we had to have it. I also learned some of the tax requirements, and all the dos and don'ts of forming and operating a business on a daily basis, which is a 24-hour, seven-day-a-week activity. This opportunity gave me a different perspective, yet it was still within my field, and it still allowed me to build on what I had learned previously.

Finally, I learned that in a business venture, the circumstances of one partner can impact the day-to-day operations and continuity of the organization. Not too long after we started the venture, Dr. Haynes received a call to return to Drew to become the President and Dean of the School. Sterling and I were so happy for him because we knew he was the best person for the job.

He and Hazel were gracious enough to leave the business in a sturdy state for me and Sterling to run, but we knew we could not carry on with just the two of us, so we finished what needed to be finished and we closed the business. By 1980, the venture had ended but not the wonderful, couple-mentoring-couple relationship with Dr. and Mrs. Haynes.

This was the only time in my career that my focus was on profit generation. It was a different type of experience than the others that I had previously enjoyed, but the lessons made me a better-rounded person, and I believe, they helped me to be more effective in my later professional endeavors. This period also provided me with a chance to be more settled and homebound, which was a blessing since in 1979, my son Aaron came along.

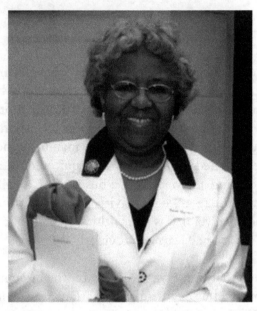

Mrs. Hazel Edgecombe Haynes (Courtesy of the Haynes Family)

Through this opportunity, I also became acquainted with the United States Agency for International Development (USAID). The contract that we were awarded allowed me to become familiar with the mechanisms and techniques involved with contracting for the federal government. Little did I know that I would soon be on the other side of the desk at USAID working with contractors to make a difference in public health.

CHAPTER EIGHT

Working with the Federal Government

By the early 1980s, a turning point was occurring. Many procedures were developing to aid the physician in the care of patients. Along with these procedural shifts came the evolution of new roles for professionals in the expanding circle of care. Rather than seeing the physician as an isolated provider, the healthcare industry was beginning to view physicians as coordinators of efforts associated with the provision of care. However, the physician was trained to depend on these services but not necessarily to incorporate recommendations into an overall care pattern or a therapeutic regimen.

In 1981, the American Public Health Association (APHA) outlined the public health role of the pharmacist in policy number 8024. "The Role of the Pharmacist in Public Health" was a pioneering statement that was later updated in 2006. The 2006 version reads, in part:

> The pharmacist's role is expanding beyond the traditional product-oriented functions of dispensing and distributing medicines and health supplies. The pharmacist's services of today include more patient-oriented, administrative, and public health functions. There are many functions of public health that can benefit from pharmacists' unique expertise that may include pharmacotherapy, access to care, and prevention services.

The 1981 policy position builds on the previous publication that I co-wrote along with Joel Kahn in 1971. I also was a co-author of the position paper in 1981 with Dr. Patricia Bush and the late Mr. Keith Johnson of the United States Pharmacopeia (USP).

A Turning Point in Health Care Delivery Services at USAID

It was against this landscape that I embarked on a new role with the federal government. The U.S. Agency for International Development (USAID) was in the early stages of addressing the World Health Organization's (WHO) Alma-Ata Declaration of 1978, "Health Care for All." The Alma-Ata Declaration was a landmark policy that identified primary health care as a key component to achieving health for all people and defined the elements of primary health care that could be adopted by member states.

According to the Declaration:

> *The Conference strongly reaffirms that health, which is a state of complete physical, mental, and social well-being, and not merely the absence of disease or infirmity, is a fundamental human right and that the attainment of the highest possible level of health is a most important world-wide social goal whose realization requires the action of many other social and economic sectors in addition to the health sector.*

One of the eight elements of the Alma-Ata Declaration by WHO was the provision of essential medicines to all people within the framework of primary health care.

With a concentrated focus on primary health care, USAID supported the building of basic facilities in countries around the world that could be staffed by a trained person from the community to handle basic health problems. They called these facilities health huts.

In 1980, I was referred by colleagues within the Black Caucus of Health Workers of APHA to USAID to work on a six-month consultancy to assist with problem solving on primary care health huts that had no drug supply. At the time, I had recently been awarded the Hildrus A. Poindexter Award by the Black Caucus of Health Workers of APHA for outstanding service in the field of health. This prestigious award recognized the work and legacy of Dr. Poindexter, a physician bacteriologist who studied tropical diseases in public health worldwide. I was the first African American female to be accorded the honor. Dr. Thomas Georges, Chief of the Office of Health in the Africa bureau at the time, played a major role in getting me involved as a consultant. He believed that with my pharmacy background, I would have a unique and valuable perspective that could help them to solve some real-world public health problems.

As an expert consultant for USAID's Africa Bureau, Health and Nutrition Division, I was assigned to travel up to eight countries in Africa in three months to conduct limited assessments and to provide expert technical and policy guidance to the Bureau on ways to effectively provide basic pharmaceuticals through funded primary health care projects. The countries I visited were: Senegal, Mali, Liberia, Zimbabwe, Ivory Coast, Gambia, and Zaire – now the Democratic Republic of the Congo. In this role, I also wrote policy and guidance documents that would help to facilitate the improved access to drug supply in these various countries.

This role was important for several reasons. For one, it helped to change the way pharmacists were seen at the time. In the past, it was not customary for pharmacists to be consulted on matters of public health. Most people just looked at pharmacists as commercial beings. They did not see that we had any health training at all. We were sellers of products, but we were not to provide information. In fact, in the late 1960s, pharmacists were prohibited from discussing certain aspects of medication use with patients. However, pharmacists are among the most accessible healthcare professionals, so it makes sense to involve them in the development of public health decisions and in the implementation of those decisions.

Each of the countries I visited had different challenges. For example, many of the countries had limited organization in their drug supply. In those regions, the people needed access to basic medicines, such as aspirin, paracetamol, or ointments for skin rashes. In other countries, only some of the people had access to essential medicines. For example, the drugs might have been in the capital city, but they weren't getting to rural locations where patients needed them.

To address these issues, a number of questions needed answers. For example, should the capital city warehouse be the deciding factor on the number and kind of drugs to be "pushed down" to the rural location? Or, should the location send requests to the capital city and in this manner "pull their supply of drugs down?" My team had to articulate those types of recommendations, as well as the issues associated with each strategy.

As part of the mission, I prepared a report on the findings from a pharmacist's point of view: "The Provision of Pharmaceuticals in Selected Primary Health Care Projects in Africa: Report of a Survey (November 1981)." This survey was followed by a set of recommendations in the report "Providing Basic Medicines in Rural Primary Health Care Projects in Africa: Technical Guidelines (1981)." We ensured its distribution, discussion, and role in program planning, implementation, and evaluation by USAID. After the initial consultancy, I received a letter from James D. Shepperd, MD, MPH, who was the director of the Africa Bureau, Health and Nutrition Division. In the letter, Shepperd applauded my work, writing:

> The area of pharmaceuticals in primary health care in Africa is one that will have long and short-term benefits from your expertise and from your comprehensive qualitative approach. Staff are presently more aware of programming possibilities in this area and have utilized many of the recommendations you provided as a technical resource.

Shepperd also shared some of the accomplishments of the assignment:

Your reports and documents will become a resource for all Africa bureau health programs. Your plan for the Liberian primary health care project will serve as a model for other similar projects. Your system of cost projection for the Regional Communicable Disease Control project has been adopted in several economic studies of health programs.

AID – Pharmaceuticals + Projects

UNITED STATES INTERNATIONAL DEVELOPMENT COOPERATION AGENCY
AGENCY FOR INTERNATIONAL DEVELOPMENT
WASHINGTON D C 20523

October 2, 1981

Dr. Rosalyn C. King
915 South Belgrade Road
Silver Spring, MD 20902

Dear Dr. King:

I would like to take this opportunity to recognize the positive contribution of your consultancy to program activities in the Health and Nutrition Division of the Africa Bureau of the Agency for International Development.

The area of pharmaceuticals in primary health care in Africa is one that will have long and short-term benefits from your expertise and from your comprehensive and qualitative approach. Staff are presently more aware of programming possibilities in this area and have utilized many of the recommendations you provided as a technical resource.

This new awareness by AID/W and USAID in Africa of the problems of pharmaceutical supply and of the availability of plans for solving these problems will make primary health care projects take on new probabilities for success. Addressing the technical aspects of this major barrier to implementation of African health programs has also given creditability to the Health and Nutrition Divisions technical support role. The numerous requests for further exposition about pharmaceutical supply systems, and for consultation on country specific and regional project problems attest to the quality of the expert technical knowledge you provided. Your reports and documents will become a resource for all Africa bureau health programs. Your plan for the Liberian primary health care project will serve as a model for other similar projects. Your system of cost projection for the Regional Communical Disease Control project has been adopted in several economic studies of health programs.

You possess a unique combination of expertise: Health Care Evaluation, Public Health and Pharmacy. And, because you were able to perform in such a professional and timely manner, you were awarded a contract to provide further technical guidance for program and policy consideration and development.

You are to be congratulated for a job well done. I look forward to equally successful performance under and completion of the contract.

Sincerely,

James D. Shepperd, M.D., MPH
Director,
Division of Health and Nutrition
Africa Bureau

The work went so well that, as a follow-on, The Bureau of Science and Technology, which housed all technical health and population policy experts at USAID, asked me to join their office. My role was to continue the work we began for the Africa Bureau and to be available to conduct problem solving, program design, program evaluation, and general consultation to the agency worldwide. Through an Intergovernmental Personnel Action (IPA), I continued as a member of the Charles R. Drew University but acted as a full-time staff of USAID.

The IPA Mobility Program provides for the temporary assignment of skilled personnel between the federal government and state and local governments, colleges and universities, Native American tribal governments, federally funded research and development centers, and other eligible organizations. Federal government employees could take assignments with these organizations without the loss of employee rights and benefits, and vice-versa. In my case, my IPA assignment had me doing work for the federal government, but I received my salary from Drew.

My IPA assignment was a three-year project that was extended for two more years until November 1985 with approval of the agency health sector council, which was composed of leaders in health policy and programs across all USAID bureaus of that time (Africa, Asia, Latin American and the Caribbean, Near East). Efforts focused on developing project frames and initiatives such as the Organization of Eastern Caribbean States Drug Procurement, which continues to this day to enable pooled procurement of drugs, and the evaluation of drug distribution systems in preparation for upgraded levels of USAID support in primary health care, among others. Here is a 1983 sample of the process of outlining requests for my input and task with timelines.

UNITED STATES INTERNATIONAL DEVELOPMENT COOPERATION AGENCY
AGENCY FOR INTERNATIONAL DEVELOPMENT
WASHINGTON D C 20523

MEMORANDUM

TO: S&T/H, George Curlin

FROM: NE/TECH/HPN, Charles N. Johnson

SUBJECT: IPA of Dr. Rosalyn King

This is to confirm our understanding on sharing the
time of Dr. Rosalyn King during the two year
extension by S&T of her IPA. As discussed, we
understand she will be made available to the NE
Bureau for some portion of the two years of her
extended IPA to assist in developing the Bureau's
initiatives in the pharmacy/pharmaceutical area.
Although we have not determined the exact amount
of time to be involved, our understanding is that
it could be up to forty weeks over the next twenty-
four months. The types of activities that Dr. King
would perform are described in the attached list.
We are prepared to be helpful in the administrative
requirements of processing her extension and during
periods she is working with us.

The Bureau is very appreciative of S&T's support for
our efforts to develop a strong field program in this
area. We feel that you have shown leadership in this
sector and look forward to working together in bringing it to fruition in the field.

Attachment: a/s

cc: S&T/H, Rosalyn King
     S&T/MGT, Margaret Thome
     NE/EMS, Alberta Talbert
     NE/DP, Robert Bonnaffon

Representative List of Activities
for IPA - Dr. Rosalyn C. King

Jordan

Provide the Jordan Mission with technical assistance to implement
recommendations itemized in the Pharmaceutical Sector Study for family
planning activity. This includes possible intermediary - funded seminar on
role of pharmacists in family planning; training; and follow-up with MOH
regarding needs in drug legislation, control and information. Time:
Approximately 4 weeks.

Lebanon

Provide technical input for mission as it considers additional activities
re: public/private sector partnership in pharmaceutical. Time: Unknown.

Egypt

In Egypt, follow-up Sector Study recommendations and provide technical
assistance in the diarrheal disease control project on the production of
ORS. Also provide an overview of the pharmaceutical aspects of the C.I.P.
program there.

Additionally, to meet with F.O.F. in follow-up to study. Time:
Approximately 8 weeks.

Morocco

Mission has expressed interest in developing activities in the Sector but
their needs are undetermined at this time. Time: Unknown.

Yemen

Assist in finalizing plans for Tihama pharmacy study as well as
"projectizing" recommendations of study. Also to monitor study and assure
integration with other potential bilateral health/population project
activities. Time: Approximately 3 weeks.

Tunisia

Assist mission in exploring feasibility of country-wide conference/seminar
related to pharmaceutical sector. Time: Unknown.

Regional

Provide technical assistance in regional population project on
use/development of point-of-purchase materials in retail sales in
pharmacies and explore ways to bring indigenous manufacturer into the
process of developing such materials. Time: 3 weeks.

On a region-wide basis, provide technical assistance in dealing with the
role of the private sector in ORT. Time: 3 weeks.

There were major lessons to be learned as I performed in this pioneering
role, as I confronted the bureaucracy and as I adjusted to the travel.

A Pioneering Role

One of my challenges was posing new ideas that health professionals had not heard before. With my background as a pharmacist, my perspective differed from what many of the other consultants and health professionals were accustomed to sharing.

There were also challenges that stemmed from being a Black woman with such a high level of responsibility. In the early 1980s, most of the consultants sent by USAID to the field were White males. It was unusual to see a female, let alone a female of color. In fact, once I was left at the airport because those who were supposed to pick me up were looking for a White man. Luckily, I was welcomed by some members of the local community, who took me to their home, offered me a home-cooked meal, and then helped me get to the local USAID office.

From that time on, I insisted on knowing where arrangements for my lodging were made, as I could always get a taxi to a hotel. However, USAID began to address the issue of diversity within its consultant pool. On a trip to Jordan in 1983, my work team included a White male and an Egyptian, Arabic-speaking female. The diversity of our team surprised many of those around us.

Just before my IPA ended, I found myself literally left at an airport upon my arrival in another country as the airport was closing. Thank goodness I knew my lodging arrangements and took the last taxi in the taxi stand to the hotel and checked in. The next morning, I called the local USAID office to let them know I had arrived and was ready for duty. They were shocked to hear from me, as the driver sent to convey me from the airport to the hotel told them that Dr. King had not arrived. After a good laugh, they sent the driver over to the hotel to pick me up. When he arrived, I was sitting in the lobby, reading. I heard a commotion near the front desk. The driver was arguing with the hotel receptionist that the person they were pointing out could not be Dr. King as he was looking for a white man! I calmly walked over to the brown-skinned man and introduced myself and asked if he was having a good day!!

71

Some White consultants would be so bold as to ask me how I managed to get such a position. They might say, "How did you get here?" I had a number of different ways to handle that type of question. Sometimes I would say, "Oh, I took a plane, or I took a train, or I drove." But the other times, when I felt that there was a greater point to be made, I outlined some of my background and how my skills were being used to help them to address the needs within the target community.

I also used the opportunity to give credit to Historically-Black Colleges and Universities (HBCUs), and emphasize the fact that they trained many capable healthcare professionals. I wanted to make sure people knew that there was a talent pool, and I was just one drop in a greater bucket of talent, even though I had not graduated from an HBCU but worked in one.

Confronting the Bureaucracy

According to Merriam-Webster, a bureaucracy is:

1. a: a body of non-elective government officials
   b: an administrative policy-making group
2. government characterized by specialization of functions, adherence to fixed rules, and a hierarchy of authority
3. a system of administration marked by officialism, red tape, and proliferation

That was indeed an accurate description of the US State Department in the 1980s. It was segmented into regional bureaus, offices, councils, technical offices, and the like, so I had to learn how to work with each section and each level within the structure. The higher the level of the entity, the fewer letters used to designate. For instance, the Secretary of State's Office was only "S."

I also had to have certain basic, fundamental principles to stand on as well. I insisted that my full title be used when in formal dialogues with colleagues and on formal documents. I used formal titles with others as well in these same settings. For instance, persons were not used to pharmacists being titled 'Dr.'. Some colleagues did not understand what a Doctor of Pharmacy was or how one was earned. It was important that I use these titles and educate people to help promote the conceptual use of the pharmacist in public health and in the overall health care system.

In many cases, creativity was needed for me to get credit for my work. In those days, when you wrote a document, whoever was the head of the unit would put his/her name on it, especially if it was a policy document. In my case, they downgraded the document from a policy document to a guidance document so I could put my name on it as the leader of a group. That was the only way I received credit for it.

During the period that I worked with the USAID, I traveled around the world and led the development of the first *Pharmaceuticals in Health Assistance* guidance document. I consulted in Egypt, Mali, Ivory Coast, Liberia, Togo, Senegal, Gambia, Kenya, Zimbabwe, Congo, Indonesia, Jordan, Yemen, Guyana, Jamaica, Barbados, St. Lucia, Grenada, Antigua, Montserrat, Dominica, St. Vincent, and the Grenadines and Switzerland at WHO. A table of travel is presented later.

Further, I was assigned project management duties. One of the projects I was assigned to manage was the Health Development Planning and Management program conducted by the School of Public Health at Johns Hopkins University and the Harvard Institute for International Development. That kept me in close relations with those universities. Later, I was asked to assist other office mates to manage the production of the MEDEX Primary Health Care Series Training Modules written by Dr. Richard Smith of the University of Hawaii John A. Burns School of Medicine.

I also represented USAID at various conferences. The World Health Organization and the Harvard University School of Public Health mounted an international conference on essential drugs, and I was the official lead and representative for USAID at that conference in 1984.

There was another conference in Alexandria, Egypt on the role of the pharmacist in family planning. It was another opportunity for me to serve as the USAID planner and representative. Providing input on the function of pharmacists was a key component to my role as planner and collaborator with many health professionals and pharmacists from many countries. It was a landmark conference for a key family planning organization in Egypt, Family of the Future (FOF).

The whole experience was helpful to me personally and professionally, and it helped to contribute to my thinking on what a pharmacist can do when incorporated into a community, primary health care, or public health effort to serve the underserved.

The experience also helped me to build on ideas and reinforced concepts that I had espoused with Joel Kahn in the 1971 paper, "The Pharmacist as a Member of the Health Team."

In this capacity, I continued to advise the work and personnel of the agency, and I developed program and policy related to issues pertaining to the supply of basic medicines and the use of pharmacy personnel. In a memorandum issued by James E. Sarn, he described the work I did as part of the USAID Agency-wide Essential Drugs Committee:

> The first activity undertaken by the Committee was the development of a document to provide guidance to the Agency on improving pharmaceutical activities in health assistance. Dr. Rosalyn C. King, an IPA from the King/Drew Medical Center in Los Angeles and a public health pharmacist working with S&T/H from November 1981 through February 1985, prepared the paper.

The Pharmaceuticals in Health Assistance Guidance document focused on strengthening the pharmaceutical sector of a country to increase access to essential drugs on the service level. Listed interventions were:

• Policy dialogue
• Use of the private pharmacist

- Improvement of logistics management
- Self-financing methods
- Operations research
- Indigenous production
- Procurement of pharmaceuticals
- Manpower development
- Drug utilization data and information

Work-related INTERNATIONAL TRAVEL (1970-2014)

	Region/Country	Pharmacy Related Work or Auxiliary Visit	Date of visa or work
		AFRICA	
1	Burkina Faso	Conference Presentation – ICASA	12/01
2	Cameroon	Drew IHI Project Dir – MOH;	6/87
		PROJET SESA	5/89; 10/89; 10/90
3	Congo	USAID PH Advisor – WHO/AFRO	4/81; 7/86
4	Democratic Republic of the Congo (Formerly Zaire)	Drew/ IHI Proj Dir –MOH,	4/81; 3/86; 7/86;
		UNIKIN; research	9/88
5	Egypt	USAID PH Advisor, program evaluation	8/82; 9/83
		FOF Conference Technical Advisor for USAID	4/83
6	Gambia	USAID & MOH; program evaluation	12/82; 3/98
7	Ghana	PACE/WAPF – conference (USAID Project)	8/01
8	Ivory Coast	USAID/REDSO – PH advisor/consultation	5/81; 4/85; 5/89;
		visit	11/09; 12/01
9	Kenya	USAID/REDSO PH Advisor;	4/81; 3/86; 5/06
		Drew Program	7/87; 11/88
		ROADS program review	2/08
10	Liberia	USAID & MOH advisor/consultation	5/81; 9/88
		Program evaluation/project design	5/81; 11/81
11	Mali	USAID PH Advisor, program evaluation.	3/81
12	Nigeria	Country introductions, familiarizations and auxiliary visits	3/81; 4/81; 5/81; 6/81; 7/87
		Project Director – GHAIN- program technical guidance and management	2004 -2008 (10 periods)
		SIDHAS – design consultation	2011
		Protocol Funeral Visit	5/2014
13	Senegal	USAID & MOH consultations; program design	3/81; 5/81; 7/86; 10/86
			11/82
14	South Africa	Auxiliary Transit Visit;	4/81
		ROADS program review	2/08
15	Swaziland	Drew/MSH IHI Project	6/87; 12/88
		Dir PHC Project– MOH;	
16	Togo	USAID representative to APHA Conference	11/81
17	Uganda	ROADS – review and meeting with officials in Busia	3/81; 5/06
			2/08
18	Zimbabwe	USAID PH Advisor/Consulting- MOH	4/81

Region/Country	Pharmacy Related Work or Auxiliary Visit	Date of visa or work
ASIA		
1 China (Hong Kong)	Transit visit	6/84; 3/09
2 Indonesia	USAID PH Advisor;	6/84
	Drew – University of Yogyakarta: Project Research;	6/86
	USAID program evaluation	10/91
3 Japan	Auxiliary visit	7/84; 11/91; 6/86
4 Singapore	Auxiliary visit	10/91
AUSTRALIA		
	Conference – 63rd FIP 2003-PACE	
MIDDLE EAST		
1 Jordan	USAID PH Advisor to MOH& program design	8/82; 4/83; 10/83
	USAID/Jordan Pharm. Assoc.	2/84; 4/84
2 Yemen	USAID – MOH; program design	9/83
NORTH AMERICA		
1 Canada	Conference – 45th FIP - DREW	9/85
2 Mexico	Conference – MOH, Johns Hopkins & Drew/ IHI	3/87
SOUTH AMERICA		
1 Guyana	USAID PH Advisor – Consulting Program Impl	12/84
CARIBBEAN		
1 Jamaica	USAID PH Advisor	1/84; 2/84
	To MOH Program Design;	
	Jamaica Pharmaceutical Society Presentation	6/94
	PACE Center Research & Presentation	1/95; 10/95
2 Barbados – USAID/HDQ with site visits to:	USAID PH Advisor to MOH Program Design for OECS	2/84
3 • St. Lucia	USAID PH Advisor & MOH Program Design	"
4 • Grenada	USAID PH Advisor & MOH Program Design	"
5 • Antigua	USAID PH Advisor & MOH Program Design	"
6 • Montserrat	USAID PH Advisor & MOH Program Design	"
7 • Dominica	USAID PH Advisor & MOH Program Design	"
8 • St. Vincent and the Grenadines	USAID PH Advisor & MOH Program Design	"

	Region/Country	Pharmacy Related Work or Auxiliary Visit	Date of visa or work
		EUROPE	
1	England	APhA Project Consulting – PSGB;	9/70
		Visit	2014
2	France	Visit	9/70
		Conference: 62nd FIP Congress 2002- PACE	9/2002
3	Germany	Transit visit	4/98; 9/95; 10/00
4	Greece	Transit visit	
5	Italy	Visit to Vatican on a layover	
6	Moldova	UMF Conference - PACE	10/98
7	Netherlands	Transit visits	11/04;05
8	Romania	PACE Center & World Vision	9/96
		PACE Center & UMF-Cluj Projects	1997 – 2002 (10 periods)
9	Russia	PACE Center Program Development;	5/95
		University of St. Petersburg, HUCE 1st CE Course abroad	4/95; 10/95
10	Switzerland	USAID PH Consulting – WHO	5/81
		USAID PH Panelist/ Burgenstock Meeting – How can the Public and Private Sectors Cooperate in Health in the Middle East	4/84

APhA = American Pharmacists Association
Auxiliary Visit = transit or approved layover
FOF = Family of the Future
FIP = International Pharmaceutical Federation
HUCE = Howard University Continuing Education
IHI = International Health Institute
MOH = Ministry of Health
MSH = Management Sciences for Health
OECS = Organization of Eastern Caribbean States
PH = Public Health
PSGB = Pharmaceutical Society of Great Britain
REDSO = Regional Office of USAID
SESA = Santé De L'Enfant du Sud et Adamaoua - Child Health in South and Adamaoua
UNIKIN = University of Kinshasa
UMF = University of Medicine and Pharmacy, Cluj-Napoca
WAPF = West Africa Pharmaceutical Federation

Adjusting to the Travel

My work with USAID was not only a professional turning point, it was also a personal one. It was the first time I had traveled to many of these countries. I was nervous, but I felt a sense of adventure. With the 91st Psalm to give me peace, I reminded myself that God created the entire world and each human in it. I found that in all cases, I had more in common with the people I interacted with than I had differences, and I accentuated the commonalities.

There was some preparation that I had to do prior to embarking on this part of my professional journey. For one, I had to learn French in order to communicate in some of the African countries I would be visiting. I would not be given an interpreter to work with, and without the ability to communicate once I got on the ground, I wouldn't be able to do my job. So, I was required to learn French up to a level 2 – a working knowledge – at the Foreign Service Institute (FSI) in six weeks. I had an intensive training every day for four hours so that I could gain the necessary level of proficiency. Some said this was unusual as most consultants were given interpreters. However, I was considered staff and therefore I viewed this as a blessing to add French to my tested knowledge of Spanish and Latin.

Another preparation was to delegate some of my "home" responsibilities as a daughter of retired parents, wife, mother, and engaged community person. Thank God I had a support circle. I had to call on my retired mother to come oversee and care for the "home and hearth" while I traveled. After all, there were two children in school and a vibrant husband that needed support. Sometimes on short trips, I would take my son to my parent's home and let my daughter and husband fend for themselves – they could and they enjoyed "father-daughter" time.

Once I arrived in an African country, getting used to the local communities was also an adjustment. Though the nationals were always very hospitable, I had to be careful with things such as eating since I had a severe food allergy and didn't eat certain nuts and fish. Additionally, I had to learn quickly to navigate the culture and not violate a taboo.

Most times I was successful but in Russia I had to be steadfast in refusing to join the local custom of some who wanted vodka with breakfast. I "invented" Dr. King's "champagne," using a commonly available seltzer water with plenty of fizz. When offered vodka, I would refer to my special champagne.

There were cultural adjustments, as well. I had to get used to talking to people who looked like me but considered me to be an outsider. I would say, "I'm an African born in America," and they would look at me and say, "You are not African." They meant one born on the continent. Yet, in all of my travels and countries visited, I did not feel as threatened because of the color of my skin as I did at home. Yes, I was an oddity, a foreigner, but not a threat.

The amount of time I spent in each country varied from one week to several months. If the visit was a consultation, I often spent a shorter amount of time in the country. This was the case for Yemen; I was there for one week to assist USAID in its collaboration with the World Bank on matters pertaining to pharmaceuticals. On the other hand, I was in Jordan for over a month with a team to study the pharmaceutical sector — with a sector emphasis on pharmacies and pharmacists and its implications for basic health care. The team was composed of Henry Coles of Family Health International (FHI); Dr. Sohair Sukkary, an Arabic-speaking consulting sociologist; and myself of USAID.

After the study was completed and published, the Jordan Pharmacists Association invited me and a second colleague, Dr. Ira C. Robinson, to address their national convention and present the results.

As an IPA, I continued to advise the work and personnel of the agency, and I developed program and policy related to issues of supply of basic medicines and the use of pharmacy personnel. In a memorandum, James E. Sarn, MD, MPH, agency director of health and population at USAID, described the work I did as the technical leader of the Essential Drugs Committee:

The first activity undertaken by the Committee was the development of a document to provide guidance to the Agency on improving pharmaceutical activities in health assistance. Dr. Rosalyn C. King, an IPA from the King/Drew Medical Center in Los Angeles and a public health pharmacist working with S&T/H from November 1981 through February 1985, prepared the paper.

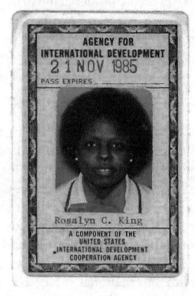

(Courtesy of the author)

MISSION FUNDS   ST/H/HSD:LRives   X5-9649

AID 5-8 (10-80)	W83-0617	AUTHORIZATION NUMBER
AGENCY FOR INTERNATIONAL DEVELOPMENT		3400081
REQUEST AND AUTHORIZATION OF OFFICIAL TRAVEL	DATE	
(See reverse of copy 8 (Employee's Copy) for Privacy Act Statement)		8 Nov 82

1. NAME AND ADDRESS OF TRAVELER	2. STATUS OF TRAVELER	3. SOCIAL SECURITY NUMBER
KING, Rosalyn C. (Pharm.D.)	☒ ADMINISTRATIVE EMPLOYEE ☐ OTHER *(Specify)* Public Health Advisor 4. OFFICIAL STATION Washington, DC	

5.
This document becomes an authorization of official travel only when the certificate of authorization has been signed by the designated authorizing officer. This travel is ordered on official business for the convenience of the government. Vouchers should be submitted promptly as provided in the applicable regulations. **MISSION FUNDS**

6.
APPLICABLE REGULATIONS: Travel and necessary expenses are authorized in accordance with the ☒ AID Handbook Number 22. ☐ Federal Travel Regulations, and the maximum per diem under these regulations is allowable unless otherwise noted in item 6.

7. ITINERARY, PURPOSE AND SPECIAL AUTHORIZATION

Travel is authorized from Washington, DC to Dakar, Senegal (30 days) and return to Washington, DC, beginning o/a November 18, 1982, and ending o/a December 17, 1982. Within country travel authorized for official business.

PURPOSE: Participation in PID Design for Phase II under Senegal Rural Health Project (685-0210).

Use of taxis is authorized while on official business.

66 lbs. accompanying baggage authorized (documents and related materials for and resulting from the study in Senegal).

Clearances: ST/HP:JJClinton   Date: 11/3/82   AFR/TR:JShepperd Date: 11/5/82
             ST/H/HSD:AHenn   Date:
             ST/H:CPease   Date: FUNDS AVAILABLE PER DAKAR 9968
                                                      dated 2 Nov 82
CABLE: DAKAR 09689
             Obligation - 5853140

8. APPROPRIATION LIMITATION SYMBOL	9. ALLOTMENT ACCOUNT SYMBOL	10. REQUESTING OFFICE SYMBOL	11. DATE
72-1131000	COEA-83-21685-U000	USAID DAKAR	11/3/82

12.
S&T/MCT, Ismaila L. Jefferson, Admin. Ofcr.   AFR/EMS, Barbara Williams, Director
APPROVING OFFICER SIGNATURE AND TITLE   OTHER REQUIRED APPROVAL

13. CERTIFICATE OF AUTHORIZATION—I CERTIFY that this authorization has been approved as indicated in item 6

Euzlear S. Foster   Deputy Chief, MO/TT
SIGNATURE OF AUTHORIZING OFFICER   TITLE

IMPORTANT Every Voucher and Message Concerning this Travel Must Refer to Authorization Number and Date at Top.

COPY FOR TRAVELER — SEE REVERSE SIDE

(Courtesy of the author)

When the IPA was finally over, James E. Sarn, M.D., MPH, USAID agency director for Health and Population wrote a letter thanking me for my service. He wrote:

You have made an important contribution in increasing the awareness and knowledge of the Agency's health professionals about the pharmaceutical sector and its role in health development. You have also built effective bridges with relevant programs domestically and internationally, such as FDA and APED. Furthermore, you have provided helpful technical guidance in our general policies and programs as well as in assisting in the design and implementation of country-specific projects. We wish you well in your future work and hope your interest and support of health development in the Third World will continue.

By this time, I was truly living my God-designed and intended purpose. I was able to bring attention to the many ways that pharmacists could contribute to public health, and I had provided input into policies and programs that were being implemented across the globe. I would continue to maintain an interest in public health across the world, and I would continue to support health development in my future roles. I was spiritually fulfilled to be utilizing my skills in the service of others.

I was pleased that Dr. Sarn noted the bridge-building work with the Food and Drug Administration (FDA). At one point during my time of service, I was called upon to clarify the product status of Oral Rehydration Salts (ORS) which were being heralded by USAID as a life-saving item to combat diarrheal disease in children under five in many developing countries. There was a need to clearly understand whether the product being promoted worldwide by USAID was classified as a food or a drug. Appropriate classification (prescription or non-prescription) would determine proper regulation and distribution. After several communications and meetings, it was determined that ORS was properly classed as a food and preliminary research on safety and effectiveness as a drug would be limited. The entire effort to get this product in the hands of many populations would have been halted had there not been this clarification. The process of the WHO Action Program on Essential Drugs (APED) also benefitted as they did not need to enter the product into a prescription or formulary status as a drug.

During all of this time, I maintained an interest in the education and development of young minority pharmacists. Opportunities allowed me to build on my first presentation during the Congressional Black Caucus Annual Legislative Weekend Health Brain Trust program in 1979. In that session, I focused on the recruitment and retention of minority students in the field of pharmacy.

In a following letter, Congressman Louis Stokes wrote:

Your testimony provided valuable information for support and initial development of health manpower legislation to be reauthorized in FY 1980. As important is a plan for built-in incentives to increase minority students in the MOD-VOPP areas as well as improve health services in manpower shortage areas.

MOD-VOPP is an acronym for the following categories of licensed, independent health professional practitioners: medicine, osteopathy, dentistry, veterinary medicine, optometry, pharmacy, and podiatry.

In 1985, the late Dr. Charles Walker, Dean and Professor of pharmacology at Florida A&M University's College of Pharmacy, asked me to become a member of the college's adjunct faculty. I served as an adjunct associate professor and was pleased because I had long held the University and its College of Pharmacy in high regard.

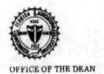

THE FLORIDA AGRICULTURAL AND MECHANICAL UNIVERSITY

COLLEGE OF PHARMACY

TALLAHASSEE, FLORIDA 32307

PHONE (904) 599-3593

OFFICE OF THE DEAN

August 9, 1985

Dr. Rosalyn King
915 South Belgrade Road
Silversprings, Maryland 20902

Dear Dr. King:

As a follow up to the previous letter of 1984, this is an official letter of appointment as an adjunct Associate Professor in the College of Pharmacy and Pharmaceutical Sciences. In this capacity, you may be asked to lecture in the following courses: (1) Clinical Practicum; and (2) Health Care Management. You may also be asked to serve as an external reviewer for grant proposals. Moreover, as in the case with Dr. Okolo, you may be involved with a FAMU faculty member on various research projects.

The details of your involvement in the above courses will be coordinated by Drs. Vernon Parker and Okolo, respectively. In regard to grant proposals, Dr. Early will contact you on a needed basis. Renumeration for the former will be at a rate of one hundred ($100) dollars per day plus expenses, while the latter will be at a rate of fifty ($50) dollars per proposal.

Please advise if additional information is needed.

Sincerely,

Charles A. Walker
Dean and Professor of Pharmacology

vbs

cc: Dr. Vernon Parker
     Dr. Okolo

B.S. Pharmacy — Doctor of Pharmacy — M.S., Ph.D. Pharmaceutical Sciences

FLORIDA A. & M. UNIVERSITY IS AN EQUAL OPPORTUNITY & EQUAL ACCESS INSTITUTION

CHAPTER NINE

Back to Drew

During my time at USAID, the Charles R. Drew University of Medicine and Science started an International Health Institute (IHI). The Institute began in 1979, under the leadership of its first director, renowned psychiatrist Dr. J. Alfred Cannon. The goal was to maximize Drew's exposure to and participation in international health. Dr. Cannon eventually moved to Zimbabwe, and the Institute was looking for someone to take over as director of the Institute with fundraising responsibilities. Subsequent candidates for the job didn't work out, and I was offered the job. But my family and I had already settled in Silver Spring, Maryland, near the Washington, D.C. area. I had no intention of leaving our home to move back to Los Angeles.

In 1986, the president of Drew, Dr. Haynes, offered me the job with the condition that Drew would put forward seed funds for an office in D.C., but I would have to raise enough revenue to make the Institute self-sufficient to do its work and cover its costs. We hired a team and together rose to the challenge so that from 1986 through 1993, the Institute was totally self-sufficient. Midway, Dean of Academic Affairs Dr. Lewis King, no relation to me, notified me that Drew conferred an associate professorship upon me in November, 1987.

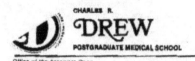

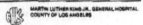

CHARLES R.

DREW

POSTGRADUATE MEDICAL SCHOOL

Office of the Associate Dean
for Faculty Affairs

KING/DREW MEDICAL CENTER

MARTIN LUTHER KING JR. GENERAL HOSPITAL
COUNTY OF LOS ANGELES

March 3, 1988

Rosalyn King, Pharm.D.
Charles R. Drew University
   of Medicine and Science
King/Drew Medical Center
Department of Family Medicine

Dear Dr. King:

On November 19, 1987, the Appointments and Promotions Committee
reviewed and recommended your appointment.

I am pleased to inform you that your appointment as Associate
Professor, I has been approved following consultation with the Board
of Directors. The effective date of your approval was January 1,
1988.

Please note on matters of compensation with regard to your appointment, you must speak to the chairperson of your department. The
Board of Directors has determined that compensation is independent of
appointment. Should there be compensation, the chairperson will, in
consultation with the Dean, decide upon a commensurate figure.
Effective dates of compensation can be only January 1 or July 1.

Again, congratulations.

Lewis M. King, Ph.D.
Dean/Vice President for
   Academic Affairs

LMK/dl

cc: Ronald A. Edelstein, Ed.D., Assistant Dean for Faculty Programs
    Ludlow B. Creary, M.D., Department Chairman
    James G. Haughton, M.D., Medical Director
    Juritta Brown, Personnel Director
    Henry Mosely, Drew Controller

1621 East 120th Street, Los Angeles, California 90059   Telephone: (213) 603-3104

I located and chose the space where the office would be, and hired the
personnel. My background with USAID was helpful because I was able
to maintain a relationship with the agency through the Institute. The
D.C. office would ultimately function as a multipurpose location to

86

facilitate all the University's D.C.-based interactions, as well as house International Health Institute staff and project personnel.

When I accepted the position, my goal was to continue to develop programs and projects for the Institute and to maintain the University's international focus by generating projects that could involve faculty, staff, and students. Working at Drew in this capacity kept me on the global health path but also made me tailor activities to the needs of the University to focus on research and service within the academic milieu.

I had to communicate my vision to others. I had to draw people around me to form teams that could help execute the projects we wanted to complete. While this was a whole new approach for me, I had ample experience collaborating with others through my work in Watts and my early days at Drew. I also now had a global perspective with some strong international relationships.

Projects Around the Globe

The International Health Institute participated in many projects around the world that made a positive difference for the people in different countries, as well as the faculty, staff, and students at Drew. Below are some of the highlights during my tenure as director from 1985 to 1993.

- The Swaziland Primary Health Care Project was intended to improve the health status of Swazi women of child-bearing age and children under the age of five. Drew partnered with Management Sciences for Health, an organization that has had a long relationship with USAID. While Management Sciences for Health managed the overall project, we handled the participant training and clinic management components of this project. A lot of things fell under this umbrella. One of the ways we aided Swaziland was by helping them to develop their formulary – the list of medications that they were going to be prescribing. Drew also provided a project manager, Mrs. F. Thomasina Paige, who handled arrangements for long- and short-term training of

Swazi students. Another contribution Drew made to the project was to maintain a full-time Clinic Management Advisor in country, Dr. Margaret Price, who helped the Ministry of Health to improve the management of clinic services.

- Project S.E.S.A. (Santé De L'Enfant du Sud et Adamaoua – Child Health in South and Adamaoua Provinces) in Cameroon was designed to help reduce the infant, child, and maternal mortality rate in that country. Drew was part of a consortium of organizations that also included The Harvard Institute for International Development and the Academy for Educational Development. Faculty from Drew helped in the planning stage of the project. Drew also provided two Maternal and Child Health Provincial Coordinators to serve in different regions of the country: Regina Dennis served in Adamaoua and Dorothy Madison-Sec in the South. These coordinators organized the training of government health workers and maintained the project management information system. Drew also provided other support in the form of a project manager, senior technical officer, and consultants. In addition, Drew contributed to the work of pro-pharmacies in Cameroon. These are non-commercial, government-sponsored entities that have a selection of essential medicines. Pro-pharmacies are typically found in rural areas where the drug supply is limited. I wrote the guidance document for the development of the project's pro-pharmacy system.

- The International Health Institute conducted pharmaceutical research through USAID's Small Research Grant Program for Historically Black Colleges and Universities. In collaboration with the University of Gadjah Mada Faculty of Medicine in Indonesia, the Institute studied the effects of the pharmaceutical rifampin. A study in Zaire conducted by Drew, The University of Kinshasa (UNIKIN) School of Pharmacy, and Florida A&M University (Dr. Eucharia Okolo) compared the concomitant use of traditional and modern medicines for the treatment of disease. The late professor and scholar Dr. Bipi Mulumba, who had been trained in medicinal and pharmaceutical sciences at the University of Buffalo, New York, was a lead collaborator at UNIKIN. Dr. Mulumba presented some of his research formally at the Drew campus in Los Angeles and presented a country flag to President Walter Leavell.

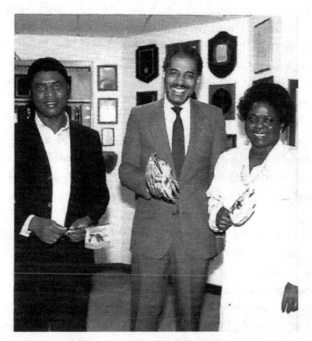

Left to Right: Dr. Bipi Mulumba of UNIKIN, President Walter Leavell of Drew, and me.

- The *Joint Memorandum of Understanding (JMOU)* was a USAID-funded program that paired Historically Black Colleges and Universities (HBCUs) with large, predominantly White schools of public health. The goal was to have the two institutions work together to plan and implement international health programs. Drew was paired with the Johns Hopkins University School of Hygiene and Public Health. The other collaborating schools were Howard University and the University of North Carolina; Meharry Medical College and Columbia University; and Morehouse School of Medicine and Tulane University. All eight of the schools participated in the International Health Network, an initiative that served as an information source to all the member institutions, USAID, and Congress.

- It was also important that we make the program useful for the students. We established and funded Drew's first international rotation for medical students, which gave them a more well-rounded education and a valuable experience.
- The first Fulbright Scholar to Drew, Dr. Ntokamunda Kadima, was a scholar and professor from the School of Pharmacy, University of Kinshasa in Zaire (now the Democratic Republic of the Congo).

While I was director, Drew celebrated the 10-year anniversary of the International Health Institute. Walter F. Leavell, MD, Drew's president at the time, wrote the following about the Institute in the program booklet celebrating the anniversary:

> *The success of Drew's international health program during the past ten years is attributable to its unique approach to international health, the quality of its leadership and the competence and compassion of the staff. In a relatively short time, the program has achieved much; providing services to twenty-five countries, initiating programs to train African physicians in public health, training physician assistants and providing overseas' experience to faculty, staff and students. It received the distinguished honor of hosting The University's first Fulbright scholar from Zaire, West Africa, under the auspices of the current Director of the International Health Institute, Dr. Rosalyn C. King and her staff, who continue the tradition of excellence begun a decade ago. Hats off to the current Institute staff and to those who went before!*

The IHI team located in Silver Spring, Maryland included, in addition to those mentioned above: Jewel Bazilio-Bellegarde, Douglas Keene, Diane Butler, Laslene Dawkins, Olga Benjamin, Lori McCray, Linda Walker and Bowyer Freeman.

Highlights Beyond Drew

In addition to my work with the International Health Institute, there were other career highlights during this time.

In 1990, I was elected to the National Committee of Revision of the United States Pharmacopoeial Convention (USPC). At that time, the USPC was the world's only private organization to set federal public drug standards. The Committee is responsible for the revision and preparation of *The United States Pharmacopoeia* and *The National Formulary*, two authoritative sources about the quality, purity, and strength of pharmaceutical drugs. USP also published the United States Pharmacopeial Drug Information (USP/DI). The Convention included representatives from schools and colleges of Medicine, Nursing, Pharmacy, Dentistry; all health practitioner professional associations and scientific bodies; state medical, dental, nursing and pharmacy societies; health consumer organizations; pharmaceutical manufacturers and their associations; governmental bodies such as FDA and state health associations, as well as invited representatives of other governments and countries. It is this collective that voted for the members of the Committee of Revision.

People

□ □

* **Bertha Watson Henry,** vice president of the Dayton chapter of the National Forum for Black Public Administrators, has been appointed assistant city administrator for Montgomery County in Ohio.

* **Jonathan Knight,** a Hallmark greeting card designer and miniatures artist, recently was inducted into the National Association Of Trade And Technical Schools Hall Of Fame headquartered in Washington, D.C.

* **Kermit R. McMurry,** director of the Nebraska Department of Social Services since 1986, recently joined the Oklahoma State Regents for Higher Education in Oklahoma City as associate vice chancellor for academic affairs.

* **Dr. Sullivan A. Welborne Jr.,** a student affairs administrator at North Carolina A&T State University in Greensboro for the past 19 years, has been named the university's vice chancellor for student affairs.

 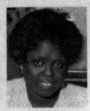 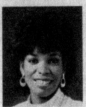 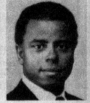

Daniel Boggan Jr. *Rosalyn King* *Kim Simpson* *Alfred Mays*

* **Daniel Boggan Jr.,** vice chancellor of business and administrative services at the University of California at Berkeley, has been elected president of the National Forum for Black Public Administrators.

* **Dr. Rosalyn C. King,** director of the Charles R. Drew University of Medicine and Science International Health Institute in Silver Spring, Md., has been elected to the National Committee of Revision of the U.S. Pharmacopoeial Convention. She is the first Black woman to hold this position.

* **Kim Simpson,** former reservations manager at The Worthington Hotel in Fort Worth, Texas, recently was promoted to Bridge manager. She will direct all food service operations on the hotel's mezzanine-level Bridge.

* **Alfred T. Mays,** vice president of research and development for Chicopee, a subsidiary of Johnson & Johnson in New Brunswick, N.J., since 1987, was appointed president of the company which develops and markets a variety of fabrics for commercial and industrial use.

20

JET Magazine, June 25, 1990, #64060, page 20

Only 114 members were selected from among 1,200 nominees and I was the first Black woman to be elected to the committee in its 170-year history. There was even a write-up about my being elected to the committee in the June 25, 1990 issue of *Jet Magazine.*

The June 25, 1990 issue of *Jet* write-up on page 20 read:

> *Dr. Rosalyn C. King, director of the Charles R. Drew University of Medicine and Science International Health Institute in Silver Spring, Md., has been elected to the National Committee of Revision of the U.S. Pharmacopeial Convention. She is the first Black woman to hold this position.*

As part of the Committee of Revision, I was chair of the International Health Advisory Panel for the publication of the USP/DI. I served in this capacity for a five-year term and was then re-elected for another five years, after which the panel was disbanded. During this time, the panel advised USP to start and strengthen its relationship with USAID, which it did and continues to this this day.

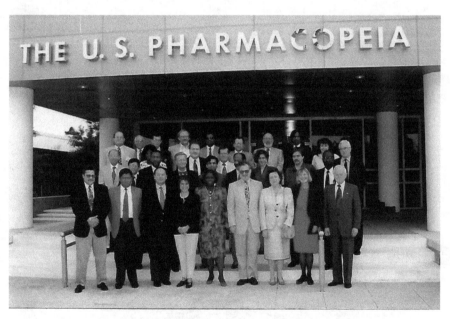

USP INTERNATIONAL HEALTH PANEL with me and Dr. Wertheimer to my left, front row, (Courtesy of the author)

In 1991, I was invited to join the National Editorial Board of the *Journal of Health Care for the Poor and Underserved.* In that role, I would be asked to review some of the submissions that would be published. In a letter welcoming me to this role, David Satcher, MD, PhD, then president of Meharry Medical College wrote:

> *I am pleased that you have accepted our invitation to join the National Editorial Board of our Journal of Health Care for the Poor and Underserved. We think strengthening the Board will greatly enhance the sophistication and power of our review process, and we are delighted that we can count on your help.*

I was proud of both of those achievements, as they allowed me to further share my unique perspective as a pharmacist with a passion for public health.

MEHARRY MEDICAL COLLEGE
OFFICE OF THE PRESIDENT

May 30, 1991

Rosalyn C. King, PharmD, MPH
International Health Institute
King/Drew Medical Center
8401 Colesville Road, Suite 303
Silver Spring, MD 20910

Dear Dr. King:

I am pleased that you have accepted our invitation to join the National Editorial Board of our *Journal of Health Care for the Poor and Underserved*. We think strengthening the Board will greatly enhance the sophistication and power of our review process, and we are delighted that we can count on your help.

While the Board represents our principal panel of reviewers, our editorial staff also relies on outside experts for advice on manuscripts that fall outside of the Board's expertise. Thus although we ask that Board members be available to review two to four papers over the course of a given year, the actual number usually falls at the low end. Kirk Johnson, editor of the *Journal*, will explain the review process further when he contacts you with an initial manuscript for evaluation. We have not planned meetings of our Editorial Board, but we do consider such gatherings to be a valuable chance to share experiences and discuss our editorial vision for the *Journal*. We will evaluate the possibility of bringing the Board together at some future point.

As you can probably imagine, launching a medical journal and keeping it afloat are no certain tasks given today's saturated publishing market. We are hopeful that our unique focus will help guarantee us a permanent niche in the market. Just the same, we would appreciate your spreading the word about the *Journal* among your colleagues, encouraging them to submit papers and to join our family of subscribers. If you would be kind enough to send us a list of colleagues or organizations you think would be interested to know about the *Journal*, we would be happy to send them a sample issue and a letter of introduction bearing your name.

We will ship you five complimentary copies of each issue of the *Journal* as it is published each quarter. Our editorial staff would be happy to send you extra copies or brochures about the *Journal* at any time should you need them.

Thank you again. We look forward to working with you in the months ahead.

Sincerely,

David Satcher, MD, PhD
President

cc: Kirk Johnson

1005 D.B. TODD BOULEVARD • NASHVILLE, TENNESSEE 37208 • (615) 327-6904/6905
FAX (615) 327-6540

The End of an Era

My experience as the director of Drew's International Health Institute was a rewarding one. In summary, the opportunity at IHI permitted me the privilege to manage and supervise the development and maintenance of technical and administrative capability for the University's international health program under a University revolving fund. IHI led the University's effort and provided technical guidance for securing a $5.3 million portfolio (grants and contracts) for technical assistance, training programs, and research in seven developing countries which helped continue the University's position as a strong collaborator in international development. Further, the office was also the designated office for the many presidential visits to Washington. However, my tenure had its share of challenges.

One of the biggest lessons I learned through my experience at the Institute was how important it is for colleagues to understand your role. When they don't, they can be the source of unfounded rumors, degradation, and speculation, especially when there is a distance separation.

I had a great, dedicated staff, and they were really working very hard. However, since my office was in D.C. (technically in downtown Silver Spring, Maryland), those who were based in Los Angeles didn't see me every day; I could not participate in the normal back-and-forth of campus life. When I would travel back to Los Angeles, I would address the faculty and share what we were doing at the Institute; I even brought collaborators from Zaire once to make a presentation about one of the research projects that we were doing there. However, office politics, financial challenges, and unsubstantiated rumors led some to question the value of what we were doing in the D.C. area, and I began to realize that some were trying to have the program moved back to Los Angeles.

This all took place at a very personally challenging time. In 1988, our daughter, Kristin, passed away. She was a third-year student at Howard University, and she had a rare form of brain cancer. The personal loss combined with the professional road bumps made this a very troubling period in my life.

Finally, in 1993, with rumored notice, Drew officials closed the D.C. office seven years after I began that portion of my career journey. I remember when we were in the process of closing the office, and people would ask, "Why are you moving?" My honest answer: "Don't ask me. Call my boss and ask him because most people thought the International Health Institute was successful under my tenure. It wasn't perfect, but it was successful."

The end of my role at the International Health Institute was a very painful time. But when the Lord closes one door, He opens another.

As the Lord would have it, I literally walked across the street and was offered a job at Howard University in its School of Continuing Education (HUCE). That would be the next chapter of my career, and a continuation of my work managing programs that would have an impact on pharmacy, pharmacists, and public health in underserved communities around the world.

CHAPTER TEN

Howard University Continuing Education (HUCE), OIP, and The PACE Center Years

Encouraging Other Pharmacists to Serve the Underserved

Howard University Continuing Education, HUCE (which, until 1996 was known as Howard University School of Continuing Education), operated across the street from the International Health Institute in downtown Silver Spring, Maryland. I was invited by Associate Dean Ponnuswamy Swamidoss to meet with Dr. Eleanor I. Franklin, who was the Dean. I shared with her my background and offered suggestions about how my experience and skills could be used at Howard. Unfortunately, later the University downgraded the School to a Program, but Dean Franklin still supported the ideas presented.

Initially, they were looking for help with structuring continuing education for practicing pharmacists in the Washington, D.C. metropolitan area. I told Dr. Franklin that I could do that, but I did not want to clash with the School of Pharmacy, which typically serves in that capacity. I suggested that the School of Continuing Education focus on taking an international approach. My suggestions were in tune with her plans for recognizing Howard's increased need to broaden its global commitment and advancement. In 1993, I began my role as the program founder and manager of the Office of International Programs (OIP). Once again, I would be focused on improving public health outcomes in underserved communities around the world. A member of the IHI team, Olga Benjamin, joined me at Howard.

OIP was designed to provide outcome-oriented training for mid- to senior-level managers and leaders from all over the world. Its purpose was to use continuing education practices and methods to create a training platform for international professionals both in the United States and abroad. Howard University has been labeled the "Capstone of Negro Education" because of its role educating generation after generation of African American students. My time heading OIP was certainly the Capstone of my career. It would be my last professional role before I retired. At OIP, I put into practice organizational development and management practices that I'd learned over the years, as well as concrete actions for getting pharmacists involved in their own transformation from sellers of products to direct contributors to patient care.

Of course, Howard had worked with the federal government in the past; however, when it came to USAID grants and contracts, interaction was limited. As a result, there wasn't a high familiarity with many of the USAID grant, contract, and cooperative agreement processes. That was an area I knew very well, and I shared my vision with the Office of Research Administration (ORA) and the School of Continuing Education about how the OIP could work with USAID as a training program contractor. Once again, my earlier career experiences provided the insight that I needed to handle the task at hand. It was as if every step prepared me for the next.

Not everyone across campus was open to my ideas at first. I literally had to convince some people to try certain strategies I knew to be approved by USAID when budgets were developed or travel was needed. In the long run, it seemed that Howard appreciated the strategies on training contracts and project development. Something must have been right.

The only serious issue was academic politics. When my training proposals were funded, the funds would be provided in the Dean's name. This might mean that the lead on a project proposal would have to take a step back as the Dean became responsible for implementing the program. This approach did not prove successful because as pitfalls arose during the implementation process, I would have to step in to get something back on track. This strategy did not continue with the latter multi-year projects.

I developed and oversaw a total of forty-four separate training and project efforts while at OIP. Each one required a relationship with a USAID official or contractor, preparation of a budget, and the recruiting and training of staff or personnel at home or abroad. We also had to prepare a proposal, negotiate the proposal to funding, set up a schedule of training, and then conduct the actual training. After each program ended, we conducted a closing ceremony and awarded continuing education certificates to participants. Finally, we ensured that Howard University received payments according to the approved training budget. Clearly, there was a lot involved with each individual project to ensure that it was a success. Individual training projects proved to be inordinately time-consuming.

Of the forty-four efforts, one was initiated with the Ralph J. Bunche Center at Howard and another with the Nigerian Institute for Pharmaceutical Research and Development (NIPRD). Nineteen were tailored training for individuals, nine were tailored trainings for groups, nine were certificate programs (for groups or individuals), and five were multi-year projects. The multi-year projects proved to be the most beneficial to the University and the overseas pharmacy community partners.

At the fifteenth anniversary of OIP in 2008, it was noted that more than 2,000 middle-to-senior level officials from twenty-seven countries and the US received training through OIP. Among the organizations and institutions that benefited: Family Health International, Nigeria's National Institute of Pharmaceutical Research and Development, and the University of Medicine and Pharmacy in Cluj, Romania. At one point, we had as many as twenty-seven staff members and twenty-four instructional faculty members. Just as I had to raise the funding for my work at Drew, I had to raise the funding for the operations of OIP. The total amount of funding generated by OIP's collective efforts from 1993 through 2008 when I retired is estimated at over $7,800,000.

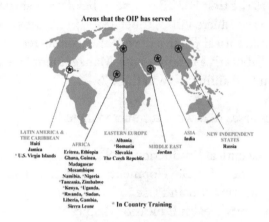

Rosalyn C. King, June 16-20, 2008, farewell presentation (Courtesy of the author)

One of the key initiatives that fell under OIP was the Pharmacists and Continuing Education (PACE) Center, a unique program that targeted the expansion of the traditional practice skills of pharmacists in developing communities abroad. I served as the founding director of the PACE Center and manager of its projects until retirement in June 2008, after which it was renamed the Pharmaceutical Care and Continuing Education Center. Dr. Grace Jennings, Christina Flood and Janine Cannon were key team members at PACE.

We developed training collaborations with several organizations including the World Health Organization, the Academy for Educational Development, the Program for International Education & Training, USAID, UNICEF, Nigeria Ports, Family Health International (FHI), and Management Sciences for Health.

I also served on Howard University Continuing Education (HUCE) management committees, such as the Management Team of HUCE, the Course Review Committee, and the Outcomes & Assessment Committee.

During my time at HUCE, I was fully responsible for project and program development. I planned and requested courses that would be given both in the United States and abroad. The course, Government Insurance Financing, was the first HUCE course to be offered abroad under direct funding. It was conducted in October 1995, in Moscow, Russia. A prior course, Pharmaceutical Security, was also conducted in Russia, but it was under collaborative funding with Management Sciences for Health as a follow-on to training here in the U.S.

Some other courses that were conducted include:

- Pharmaceutical Production
- Management for Development: Instructional Series
- Drug Information and Use
- Community Health Education Topics
- Financial Management and Pricing
- Enhancing the Mental Health of Women
- Management: Principals and Techniques of Fundraising
- Fundraising & Financial Management
- Community Medicine Topics
- Enriching the Services of Pharmacists in Health Care Delivery
- Pharmaceutical Sector Management
- Retail Pharmaceutical Purchasing
- Public Administration for Municipal Development
- Decentralized Budgeting and Financing
- Pharmaceutical and Cosmetic Quality Assurance
- Control of Management and Welfare Benefits
- Business Education Study Tour
- Management Skills and Practices

The early days saw PACE as a center for collaboration with training brokers who worked with USAID such as PIET (Program for International Education and Training). We structured programs for pharmacists and managers who wished to expand their skills and who received training support through the country offices of USAID.

But the level of human resource input was not maximized, and a way was sought to work smarter not harder. Projects that lasted longer than a few weeks or a month would do that.

Pharmacists Involvement in Primary Health and HIV/ AIDS Care

TrainPharm Project

One of the first multi-year effort partnerships was, a USAID mission-funded collaboration with the "Iuliu Hatieganu" University of Medicine and Pharmacy in Cluj-Napoca, Romania that resulted in the TrainPharm Project. Under this partnership, *Training Pharmacists for Expanded Roles in Primary Health,* we trained 1,000 community pharmacists to focus on being an agent of care rather than merely a manager of drug distribution. In Romania we collaborated on four separate projects during the period between 1996 and 2002. The first was a consultation with World Vision on Primary Health Care in Romania – joining with the Department of Family Practice in the College of Medicine at Howard. The remaining three were the Child Health Project (February 1998- June 1999) and two phases of the TrainPharm project (I: July 1999 – July 2000; II: August 2000 – July 2002). Key in-country collaborators were Dr. Marius Bojita, Vice-Rector of the "Iuliu Hatieganu" University of Medicine and Pharmacy in Cluj-Napoca, and Dr. Felicia Loghin, Professor and later Dean of the College of Pharmacy in Cluj-Napoca.

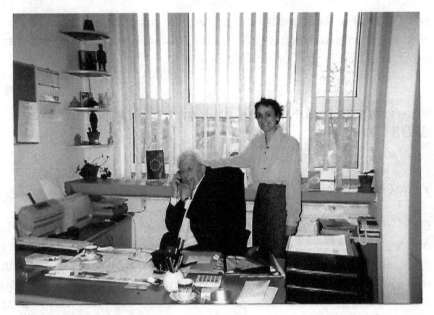

Dr. Marius Bojita, Vice-Rector and Dr. Felicia Loghin, Professor and, later, Dean. (Courtesy of the author)

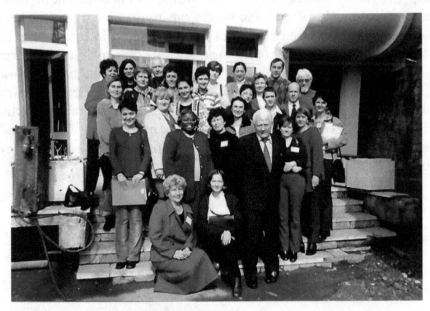

Training of Trainers, 1999 (Courtesy of the author)

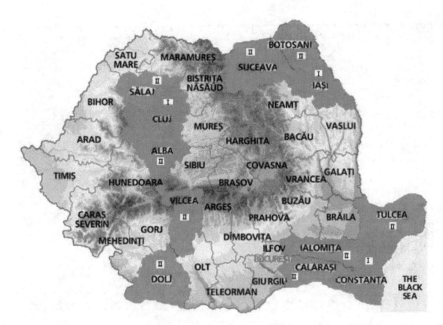

Judets of Romania whose pharmacists participated in TrainPharm I and II. (CAPSULES Vol 4, No. 1 Spring 2003, TrainPharm Project Final Report)

In recognition of the collaboration and its significance, the University Senate University of Medicine and Pharmacy in Cluj-Napoca voted to award me the title, "Visiting Professor," one of two honorary titles they award. In an investiture ceremony, I was gowned with University regalia before delivering the investiture lecture.

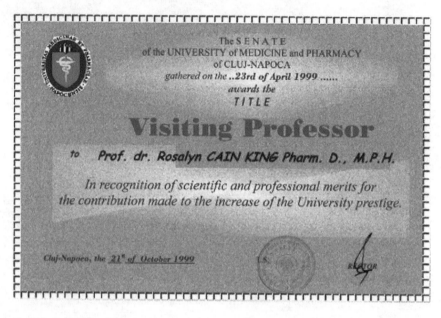

The S E N A T E
of the UNIVERSITY of MEDICINE and PHARMACY
of CLUJ-NAPOCA
gathered on the ..23rd of April 1999 ......
awards the
T I T L E

Visiting Professor

to **Prof. dr. Rosalyn CAIN KING Pharm. D., M.P.H.**

*In recognition of scientific and professional merits for
the contribution made to the increase of the University prestige.*

Cluj-Napoca, the _21^ of October 1999_   L.S.   RECTOR

(Courtesy of the author)

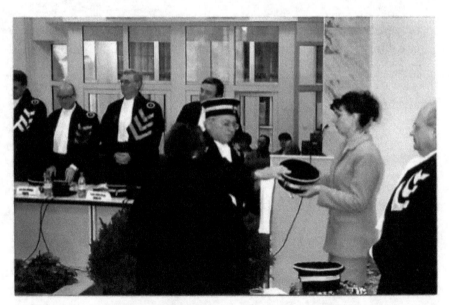

*Investiture Gowning as Visiting Professor of the University of Medicine and Pharmacy
at Cluj-Napoca, Romania, 1999. (Courtesy of the author)*

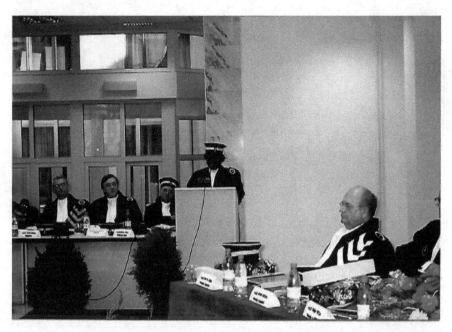

Investiture Lecture as Visiting Professor of the University of Medicine and Pharmacy at Cluj-Napoca, Romania, 1999. (Courtesy of the author)

Each local training under the project partnership had a closing ceremony and the project closed in 2002. The PACE newsletter, *CAPSULES Vol 4, No. 1 Spring 2003*, issued a special final project report.

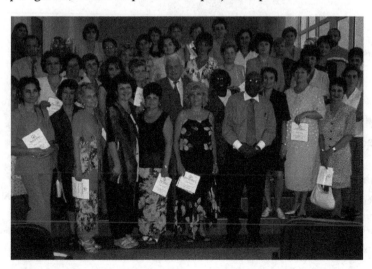

Closing ceremony, TrainPharm Project, 2002 (Courtesy of the author)

TRAIN PHARM PROJECT

Extinderea Rolului Farmaciştilor
în Asistenţa Primară de Sănătate

Organizat de Universitatea de Medicină şi Farmacie
" Iuliu Haţieganu " Cluj Napoca şi Howard University
din Washington DC - USA în colaborare cu USAID

Festivitate de închidere a proiectului

RM. VÂLCEA - ROMÂNIA
12 IULIE 2002

Organizator - Colegiul Farmaciştilor Vâlcea

Signage in pharmacies in Vâlcea România (Courtesy of the author)

The Anglophone West Africa Pharmacists HIV/AIDS (AWAP) Project

In the early days of international attention to the pandemic of HIV/ AIDS, The Anglophone West Africa Pharmacists HIV/AIDS (AWAP) Project was a study conducted from September 2000 to June 2001, with the West Africa Pharmaceutical Federation (WAPF) and PACE. At that time, WAPF consisted of the five anglophone countries: Nigeria, Ghana, Liberia, Gambia, and Sierra Leone. WAPF was founded under the leadership of its first president, Mrs. Clavenda Bright Parker, the first female pharmacy chain owner of Liberia, who some called "The First Lady of Pharmacy in West Africa," who was also a stalwart colleague at OIP. The project focused on strengthening the ability of pharmacists to provide HIV/AIDS prevention information and referral services in the region. The program ran under the premise that pharmacists were well-suited to provide information, education, and counsel to health consumers – something I had long believed in. The study was funded by USAID and later served as one basis for PEPFAR (President's Emergency Plan for AIDS Relief) work. An important outcome of this work was the recommendation generated at the final project meeting in Accra, Ghana. The ACCRA RECOMMENDATION, was in the final report but not highly published by the countries of the WAPF. The 2001 Accra Recommendation read:

- *The community **pharmacist** is a recognized health professional contributing to a favorable health outcome; and*
- *The community **pharmacy** is a patient contact site, a health service outlet close to the population which can be a fulcrum for improved health status of a community.*

This recommendation was later affirmed by WAPF at its meeting in Burkina Faso in 2001 at the 12th International Conference on AIDS and STD in Africa (ICASA), in which the work of AWAP was presented.

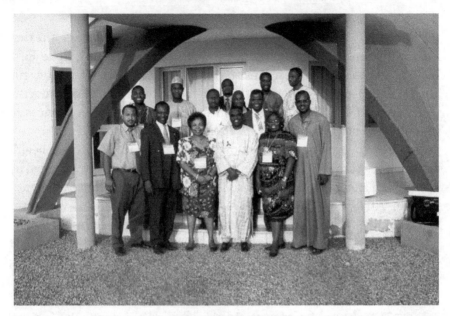

Member Representatives of the West African Pharmaceutical Federation with Mrs. Clavenda Parker (third from left in front) and me (fifth from left in front) in Burkina Faso, 2001. (Courtesy of the author)

The work of this project provided a foundation for later efforts at PACE for work in PEPFAR. The global HIV/AIDS epidemic has been one of the biggest public health crises of the last few decades. PEPFAR is a landmark United States governmental initiative that began in 2003 to address the global HIV/AIDS epidemic and help save the lives of those suffering from the disease, primarily on the African continent.

One of the highlights of my Howard University time was the opportunity to lead HUCE's collaboration with USAID missions and contractors, via the PACE Center, to implement three key programs under PEPFAR funding.

GHAIN Project

In collaboration with Family Health International (FHI), our first PEPFAR project, *The Global HIV/AIDS Initiative Nigeria (GHAIN)* project, was funded through USAID who designated it as a flagship project.

The project sought to provide HIV/AIDS services to the people of Nigeria. The GHAIN project also has particular importance for the pharmacists who work in the country because they said it rescued them from marginalization. The GHAIN project allowed them to have a more central role in what was happening in projects related to healthcare. Pharmacists were recognized as contributors over and above the selling of drug products. With this focus on pharmacy, and because this was such a critical project under PEPFAR, I am particularly proud of the work that the PACE Center was able to do in support of the GHAIN project. That work also began in 2004 under the in-country lead of the late Dr. Uford Inyang, an HU alumnus; Pharmacist Eno Ebok- Udom; and Dr. Dorothy Oqua, who is still the team leader and now the Howard University Country Director in Nigeria. Specific objectives of the Pharmacy component of the GHAIN project were to:

- enhance the use of the pharmacy as a resource center for prevention, treatment, care, and support activities for HIV/AIDS;
- advance the skills of pharmacists and pharmacy personnel in public and private sector to reduce incidence of HIV/AIDS; and
- mobilize public and private pharmacies to expand their involvement through improved referrals to HIV care and treatment sites, HIV prevention education, community education on OI, TB and ARV therapy, and adherence education for HIV infected clients.

HU-PACE strategies for achieving its objectives involved sensitization and mobilization of key persons in the Pharmaceutical Society of Nigeria (PSN), the Pharmacists Council of Nigeria (PCN), the National Institute for Pharmaceutical Research and Development (NIPRD), the National Agency for Food and Drug Control (NAFDAC), and the Food & Drugs Division of Federal Ministry of Health through a launch of the pharmacy component of GHAIN.

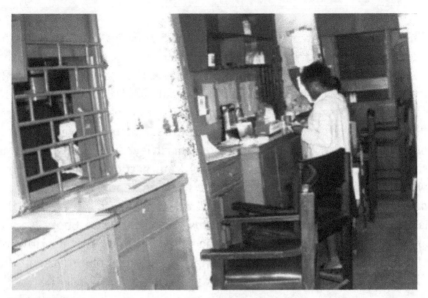

Traditional window dispensing system (GHAIN support to HIV-related pharmaceutical services in Nigeria: End of Project Monograph, 2011) (Courtesy of the author)

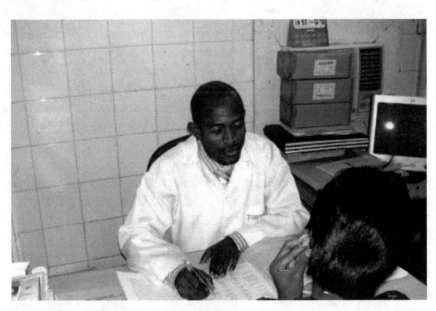

Direct pharmacist–to–patient communication
(GHAIN SUPPORT TO HIV-RELATED PHARMACEUTICAL SERVICES IN NIGERIA: END OF PROJECT MONOGRAPH, 2011)

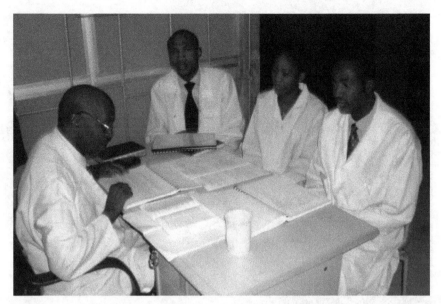

Dr. Obiaga's on-site pharmacist training for the installation of pharmacy best practices
(GHAIN SUPPORT TO HIV-RELATED PHARMACEUTICAL SERVICES IN NIGERIA: END OF PROJECT MONOGRAPH, 2011)

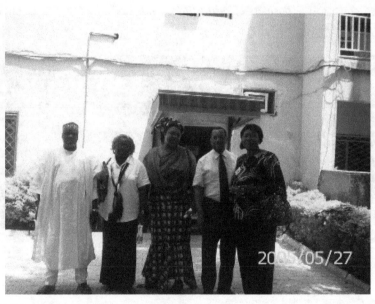

Site Visit to KANO: The Project Coordinator Dr. Grace Jennings (center) with (L to R) Pharmacists Ahmed Yakasai, Rosalyn C. King, Earnest Johnson, and Eno Ubok Udom. (Courtesy of the author)

113

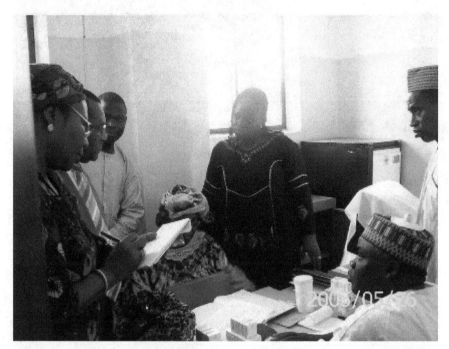

Getting down to the business of restructuring with staff in KANO. (Courtesy of the author)

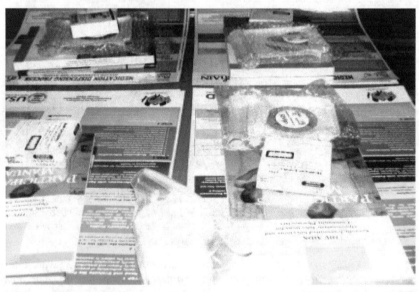

Job aids produced for GHAIN (GHAIN support to HIV-related pharmaceutical services in Nigeria: End of Project Monograph, 2011) (Courtesy of the author)

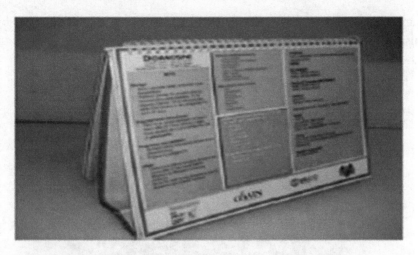

Desktop Quick Reference on Drugs for HIV/AIDS management (Drug page)

Desk top cue cards for pharmacist consultations prepared by Dr. Chris Keeys and his Clinical Pharmacy Associates team. (Courtesy of the author)

ROADS Project

The second endeavor, the *Regional Outreach Addressing AIDS through Development Strategies* (ROADS 1) project, funded by USAID, sought to reduce the transmission of HIV and improve care along major transport corridors of East, Central, and Southern Africa through nine countries There were five focus countries: Kenya, Ethiopia, Rwanda, Tanzania and Uganda. Burundi, Djibouti, DRC and South Sudan are non-focus PEPFAR countries.

Through a partnership with Family Health International, we began work on that project in 2005 under the direct, field regional supervision of pharmacist Dr. Henry Fomundam, another Howard University alumnus. The project developed some twenty-six SafeTStop sites along the transport corridors and Howard was responsible for training their pharmaceutical shop personnel in HIV prevention, care and treatment. At the time of the mid-term assessment in 2008, the project noted 302 persons trained. These staff served not only truckers on the route but also community members who turned to these sites as a first line of care.

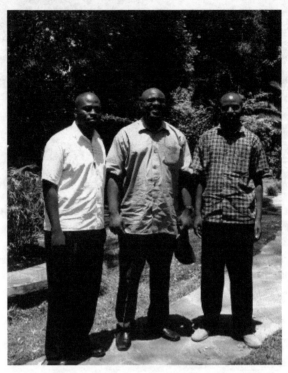

ROADS staff: Andrew Maranga, Dr. Henry Fomundam, Fred Oyaro (Courtesy of the author)

Ethiopia – The Twinning Project

Begun in Ethiopia in October, 2007, The Twinning Project was the third initiative. It was conducted in partnership with the American International Health Alliance. Our goal was to improve pre-service education by strengthening the curricula in order to support and enhance indigenous pharmacy education. This enhancement increased Ethiopian pharmacists'ability to make contributions to the fight against HIV/AIDS. That project was designed to be implemented with our School of Pharmacy, and it has continued under their auspices to this day.

At one point, there were thirty staff members overseas and four in OIP's main office dedicated to sustaining the ROADS and GHAIN projects while at the same time proposing new projects. These projects all involved training pharmacists to provide better services to those who were impacted by HIV/AIDS. By the time I retired in 2008, it was noted that more than 1,200 pharmacy or drug shop personnel in West, Central, and East Africa had enhanced their knowledge base of HIV/AIDS through the PACE Center.

There were many other projects we participated in. Here is a sampling:

OIP/PACE also collaborated with the St. Petersburg Chemical Pharmaceutical Institute in Russia. Collaboration began with two faculty members coming to USAID–sponsored training at PACE. The 1995 plan was to continue in collaboration with faculty and students from both Howard and St. Petersburg to engage in exchange opportunities. In the end, this collaboration did not happen because the Russian-speaking colleague from Howard University who would serve as staff person passed away.

OIP/PACE also received a 2004 APhA Foundation Practitioner Innovation grant that helped to support the creation of a landmark program in 2004 termed *A Dialogue: Pharmacists & Pharmacy Leadership: Making a Difference in Global Health.* The program—conducted with the mentorship of a Remington Medalist, the late Dr. Gloria Francke—convened major pharmacy organizational leadership to discuss the role of pharmacists in global health for the first time. Attendees included Dr. Nils Daulaire, then president of the Global Health Council, as well as representatives from the following organizations: American Society of Health-System Pharmacists, American Pharmacists Association Foundation, International Pharmaceutical Federation/Pharmabridge, American Association of Colleges of Pharmacy, United States Pharmacopeial Convention, Program for Appropriate Technology in Health (PATH), Management Sciences for Health, Nigerian Ports Authority, USAID, the Medical University of South Africa, the University of Maryland, Howard University College of Pharmacy, and University of Medicine and Pharmacy in Cluj-Napoca, Romania.

When we celebrated OIP's 15ᵗʰ year anniversary in 2008, several people who had participated in its programs shared their thoughts.

Mrs. Ngozi "Stella" Obikili, a pharmacist in Nigeria who attended a six-week training program in 1995, as well as trainings in 2004 and 2007, through the PACE Center, said her work benefited immensely.

> *We got exposed to a lot of things we did not know about," she says. "When we got back, we were able to introduce a lot of things that factored into our treatment.*

Dr. Felicia Loghin, who was Dean of the Faculty of Pharmacy at the University of Medicine and Pharmacy in Cluj, Romania, at the time, said:

> *We had an exceptional collaboration under the TrainPharm Project. It was very beneficial for our University and also for Romania because we managed to train nearly 1,000 pharmacists in the program.*

Global Health Experiential Externship

While at Howard, the College of Pharmacy accepted our proposal to "Expand the Boundaries of Pharmacy Education Globally with an International Health Clerkship for Students." This became the PACE Global Health Experiential Externship with Howard's College of Pharmacy beginning in 1997. Over the next ten years, eight students as well as one Hollingsworth Scholar from the University of North Carolina College of Pharmacy, were introduced to pharmacy in global health concepts and practices. The first overseas Pharmacy Extern was the late Dr. Sean Boynes, who went to Romania along with a student from the College of Medicine, Dr. Danielle Snyderman. Dr. Tatiana Bangudi was the first extern who later became employed on a project. Extern topics included:

- Physician-Pharmacist Interface in Primary Health Care in Romania
- Counterfeit Drugs in Nigeria
- The Fight Against HIV/AIDS in Ethiopia and the Pharmacist's Role in It
- Field Experiences in the Global HIV/AIDS Nigeria (GHAIN) Program
- AFRICARE and its Involvement in Primary Health Care

Here is a description of the program after two years:

THE TWO-YEAR RECORD per Tatiana Bangudi:

As of August 2001, the PACE Center has conducted two externships with the first internship occurring during the five week period of June 6, 2000 through July 7, 2000, and the second July 2 through August 3, 2001. Both have been implemented under the auspices of the TrainPharm Project. The Howard University pharmacy student in the inaugural clerkship rotated through the PACE Center for a five-week period during the student's senior year clerkship schedule. The program provided exposure to the full scope of the TrainPharm project, permitted a desk comparison of the practice of pharmacy in both the United States and Romania, called for the student to visit at least one local office of an international non-governmental agency with a focus on reproductive health to explore the breadth of their projects and determine the involvement of pharmacists, if any, and to prepare two selected bibliographies on international reproductive health articles, which addressed pharmacists' participation and/or social marketing with pharmacist assistance. At the end of the rotation, the student had to prepare two newsletter articles on the experience. The Metropolitan Washington D.C. area was the locale for the entire rotation.

Retirement

I retired from Howard University in 2008. After retirement, colleagues from Nigeria sent notes of appreciation to the University for my work with them. The following is a compilation of some of their quotes:

Dr. King contributed significantly to opening the door for pharmacists to participate in public health programs as well as inclusion of distinct pharmacy component in public health programs. More so, she contributed in widening the scope of practice of community pharmacy, showcasing their unique position in the health care terrain for implementing population level health care interventions.

--Peter Agada, Senior Pharmacy Specialist, HUGIN, Cross River State, Nigeria

"Dr. Rosalyn King changed many things in Pharmacy Practice in Nigeria during the time she worked there. She gave Pharmacy a new look and Pharmacy Profession a respect in all parts of the world. We are proud of her and wish her the best in her retirement."

--Godfrey Obiaga, Mississauga Ontario Canada

"Dr. Rosalyn King is an enigma. She is pharmacy personified. I met her a couple of times, I think twice, and participated in profuse discussions with her in the formative years of her pet project in Nigeria. She was intellectually sound, professionally competent, has excellent leadership qualities, and <was> ecclesiastically humble. In my opinion, her greatest contribution to pharmacy in Nigeria was to make pharmacists believe in themselves and to make them create an aura of professionalism that stands them out as key stakeholders in the business of healthcare delivery. Her project made the contributions of pharmacists unique, extraordinary, and

hugely beneficial to both the citizens and of course to the image of the pharmacy profession. She basically redefined the logic of pharmacy practice and the role pharmacists can play in healthcare delivery, especially at the community and primary healthcare levels.

"At the time of her retirement, she had succeeded in leaving behind an enviable and unforgettable legacy. I still remember her vividly and I feel proud and happy that her legacy is well sustained through the efforts of all key stakeholders in the project. I am confident that those who worked more closely with her will speak more on her sterling qualities. She certainly has been a blessing to the pharmacy profession and to mankind. God bless and keep her in good health today and always."

-- Joel E.B. Adagadzu, FPSN, FPCPharm.,
Chief Consultant, PHI Consult Limited,
Abuja - Nigeria

"Dr. Rosalyn King directed the first effective programme that led to the mobilization of Pharmacists, Pharmacy staff, and other resources of Pharmacy in the fight against HIV/AIDS in Nigeria. Dr. King is a teacher/trainer per excellence and she was instrumental in creating a pool of skilled and talented professionals who are today celebrated beyond pharmacy.

"Working through her pet project, Anglophone West African Pharmacists HIV/AIDS project and the Howard University project in PEPFAR/GHAIN, Dr. King broke several barriers especially as relates to doctor/pharmacists relationship by creating a cache of pharmacists with demonstrable skills and knowledge to contribute to the team efforts in managing the challenges of HIV/AIDS.

"Dr. King is a first-class manager of men and material with excellent interpersonal skills and an elastic capacity to positively influence anybody she comes in contact with.

"It is instructive to note that she was teacher, trainer, and mentor to at least two Pharmacists who later emerged as Presidents of the Pharmaceutical Society of Nigeria. Dr. King is a great fighter for cause of Pharmacy and Humanity. She certainly earned herself a seat in the front row of those who influenced Pharmacy practice in Nigeria and across the West African sub region."

**--Azubuike Okwor, Past President,
Pharmaceutical Society of Nigeria
& African Pharmaceutical Forum**

"Dr. Rosalyn King is a global and visionary leader of Pharmacy. Her commitment and vision led her to set up, in 1993, the Pharmacists and Continuing Education (PACE) Centre at Howard University. Through projects she implemented as the Director of the PACE Centre, she has contributed tremendously to the achievement of significant improvements in pharmacy practice in several countries across the world.

"In Nigeria, Dr. King has been instrumental to bringing significant changes in pharmacy practice in hospitals and community pharmacies across Nigeria. She spearheaded the involvement of pharmacists in public health and specifically the growth of patient focused care in pharmacy practice in Nigeria.

As Director of the PACE Centre at Howard University and a member of the FHI led consortium implementing the Global HIV AIDS Initiative Nigeria (GHAIN) project, Dr. King spearheaded the inclusion of a specific pharmacy component in the design of the GHAIN project. Under her leadership, the GHAIN project served as a platform that highlighted a specific clinical role for both hospital and community pharmacists in the prevention, treatment, care, and support of people living with HIV/AIDS as well as their families in Nigeria. The GHAIN project, which was the largest PEPFAR funded HIV program, served as a platform to strengthen pharmacy systems and services and enable other clinicians to acknowledge the clinical role of the pharmacists in the multidisciplinary health team, beyond drug procurement and supply chain management, a feat which has changed pharmacy practice in Nigeria.

"The accomplishments by the Howard University-PACE Nigeria Team under Dr. King's exemplary leadership has continued after her retirement in 2008. Her vision has been sustained in the Sustaining Comprehensive HIV/AIDS Response through Partnership (SCHARP) program funded by CDC and the Strengthening Integrated Delivery of HIV/AIDS Services (SIDHAS) program funded by USAID. These programs have further strengthened the unique and critical role of the community pharmacy as a first point of contact for clients seeking care. These public health programs have served as platforms to expand the role of pharmacists in HIV/AIDS and TB health care delivery in Nigeria to include not just the provision of pharmaceutical care and drug inventory management, but also the provision of pharmacy based HIV Testing Services, TB screening and linkage to care, and pharmacists' supervision of primary health care centers without adequate human resource. The role of the Lady Pharmacist as a resource for interventions on issues faced by women, adolescents, and children infected or affected by HIV/AIDS has been promoted.

"Additionally, as part of the pharmacist's contributions to the attainment of HIV epidemic control in Nigeria, private sector community pharmacies are being linked to public hospitals to serve as satellite pharmacies that provide routine drug refill services, adherence monitoring, and chronic care screening to *stable clients, another feat, which was hitherto unknown in the Nigeria health sector.*

"The pharmacists and peoples of Nigeria will always remain grateful to Dr. King for her vision and commitment to the tenets of lifelong learning for pharmacists for the health of all mankind."

--Dorothy Oqua Ph.D., FPC Pharm.
FPSN Country Director,
Howard University Global Initiative Nigeria"

In recognition of these and other sentiments, as well as for serving as Chair of their 2006 annual convention, the Pharmaceutical Society of Nigeria presented me with their award of appreciation of service in 2006.

After my retirement, I continued to consult for the PACE Center from 2008 to 2011. It allowed me to continue to be an advocate for advancement in international health care while promoting the idea that pharmacists are an asset when it comes to public health.

I have continued to work as a consultant from time to time and have been blessed with the opportunity to continue my advocacy for pharmacists. For example, in 2018, I agreed to do two case studies on Romania and Nigeria, respectively, with in-country collaborators. In both studies, I described how changes to pharmacy education and training in those countries have contributed to a shift from the image of pharmacists as pill dispensers to pharmacists playing a larger role in helping improve public health. The case studies were published in the chapter "Dynamic Relationship Between Education, Regulation and Practice: Case Studies and Examples" in the *Encyclopedia of Pharmacy Practice and Clinical Pharmacy*, published in 2019.

I am proud of the lessons I learned and the impact we made during my time at HUCE and the PACE Center. Through the work we did, we served global populations, supported Howard University's leadership status in the global arena, and made some contribution to the positioning of HUCE for growth. We also learned how to make project-based training more efficient and effective, and we leveraged project alliances to make a greater impact.

I will always consider my time at Howard University to be one of the highlights of my career, and I am thankful for the profound professional and spiritual impact God privileged me to have on His Children.

CHAPTER ELEVEN

Spirituality and My Journey

I can't write the events of my journey as a pharmacist without also including the impact of my spiritual life. Religion and spirituality have always been important to me. My faith fueled my decision to become a nun, and though I left the convent, it continued to play a major role in my life. I joined Mt. Calvary Baptist Church in Rockville, Maryland with my family in 1977 under the late Reverend Houston G. Brooks and was asked by Reverend Brooks to organize a women's group called United Women and make sure it was aligned with the American Baptist Churches of the South (ABCOTS).

When I took on the role, my objective was simply that the other women would accept my leadership, be encouraged, and we would band together around a common goal of "Women: Worshipping, Working, and Witnessing." However, the reaction was mixed. Some women accepted it, some balked and questioned the need, and still others did not want to gather around with "a bunch of women."

During this time, I learned how to make myself clear and translate what I had learned as a nun to Mt. Calvary. For example, I had gained a lot of experience participating in retreats when I was a nun. I was able to translate this knowledge to the women's group when we planned our first spiritual retreat.

This experience taught me that God can use a willing vessel readily, which is a lesson that I applied not only to my spiritual life but to my professional life. I also learned that we all have our own purpose, and we must learn to be sure that what we're doing in life is in alignment with that purpose.

In addition to forming the women's group, I served as a Deaconess at Mt. Calvary. I was consecrated in 1979 after a vote of the church. Just before that my daughter Kristin had become a Junior Deaconess.

As a Deaconess, it was my duty to assist in serving the spiritual needs of the church, especially during Communion service and through visits with the sick and shut-in. A Deaconess is ready at all times for prayer and service. In order for me to accomplish everything that I wanted to get done, I had to learn how to manage my time wisely. In fact, one of the most valuable lessons I learned from the experience was that enthusiasm overdone can lead to burnout!

My work as a Deaconess also gave me a better understanding of the spiritual needs of others as they moved through everyday challenges and trials. That understanding was something that I was able to apply to my career. It gave me insight into what people were going through so that I could better understand how pharmacists could improve the health and welfare of the underserved.

As my faith played such a big part of my life, it's not surprising that I would marry a man who also had a spiritual calling. My husband, Sterling King, Jr., was ordained to the gospel ministry in 1982 at Mt. Calvary. He went over to Macedonia Baptist Church in Bethesda to "help out" in 1984. The children and I would follow for selected services. He was asked to become the Assistant Pastor in 1986 and then he was installed as Pastor in 1988 after the incumbent Pastor retired. He served as Pastor for twenty-eight years and retired in 2016.

This church, located on a major thoroughfare in Bethesda, Maryland, was the last remnant of a strong African American community that had been overtaken by development when the area turned into a "wealthy" community.

When I found myself in the position of Pastor's wife, my first thought was, 'What have I gotten myself into!' However, I became comfortable in the role and worked to contribute to the growth and strength of the congregation as best I could. I contributed to the Deaconess Board, provided guidance and mentorship to the youth of the church, and played a role in church beautification activities, such as supporting a member who brought about the installation of stained-glass windows. I also served as a writer and editor for the church newsletter. This experience helped me to be a well-rounded person and gave me another outlet to devote my skills and energy.

I believe having a spiritual foundation helps you take stock of your life and determine what's most important to you as you serve your Creator. You can learn a little bit about who you are from self-development books, tapes, and theories, but there is a structure that has existed for quite a long time that a lot of people have benefited from – the theology of the Bible. While I don't have statistics to prove that theory, I can see it in the lives of people who have a scriptural foundation.

For me, my involvement in the church was a strong lesson in prioritizing. But the lessons in service and compassion helped me to be a better healthcare professional even more and influenced my ideas on how pharmacists can play a major role in public health and the overall well-being of a community.

And so, throughout this journey as a Pharmacist, I was also a Pastor's wife, Deaconess, and Sister in Christ.

CHAPTER TWELVE

A Career Path of Service –
A Legacy to Pass On

Over the course of my career I have seen the world's view of pharmacists change from serving as "pill dispensers" to contributing to the overall health of local communities with a greater focus on achieving health outcomes. I am proud to have been a part of that flow of events and in some manner contributed to that shift. I am also grateful for the opportunities I had to help promote better systems and policies that could improve the health and the lives of the underserved around the world.

In the early days of my career, pharmacists were not looked to for the wealth of information we had received during our education. We weren't given the opportunity to serve on the front line of public health. Today, pharmacists are viewed as key providers of public health support. For example, the American Public Health Association, a leading public health professional organization, has finally recognized pharmacy as one of its sections after the hard work of many, many of its pharmacist members over the years.

Many of the projects I worked on helped to bring about this change. For example, the AWAP, GHAIN, and TrainPharm projects helped to expand the role of pharmacists across the globe. My contribution to the 1971 article, "The Pharmacist as a Member of the Health Team," also encouraged an open mind about what a pharmacist could do. That article had an influence on the APHA statements on the role of the pharmacist in public health in 1981 and 2006. I'm also proud of the dialog among top pharmacy leaders that my team at the PACE Center opened up during the landmark program in 2004 called, "Pharmacists & Pharmacy Leadership: Making a Difference in Global Health."

In addition to my work advocating for pharmacists, I also believe it is important to open the door, keep it open, and prepare the next generation of pharmacy leaders. We need a pipeline of pharmacy professionals, particularly in the African American community. We also need to make sure that there are pharmacists who are dedicated to improving public health, reducing health disparities, and in general, serving the underserved in a culturally competent and compassionate manner.

To help ensure this pipeline, I started an endowed scholarship through the National Pharmaceutical Association Foundation for graduates and alumni of Howard University's School of Pharmacy who want to go into public health. My hope is that it offers some encouragement to pharmacists who want to matriculate into a public health academic setting. I chose Howard because that is where I spent a good portion of my career.

Additionally, it was amazing to collaborate with others who were willing to demonstrate interest as we explored together the idea of pharmacists working in global health projects. Those collaborations and opportunities included:

- Dr. Peggy Berry, Director of Continuing Education at Howard University
- Dr. Chris Keeys, the owner of Clinical Pharmacy Associates, an organization based in Laurel, Maryland, that provides clinical pharmacy services for hospitals. I asked him to develop a drug information packet for HIV drugs during my work on the

GHAIN project. He did a wonderful job. His organization was also a training collaborator for PACE.

- Regina Carson, a former faculty member at Howard's School of Pharmacy, who went with me to Romania several times, coauthored one of the training manuals, and served as a preceptor to a Howard College of Pharmacy student in Romania.
- Dr. Ira Robinson, a retired dean from Howard's School of Pharmacy, who wrote the first USAID formulary. He was contracted to work on the project when I worked at USAID.
- Noreen Teoh, who worked with me to organize and implement the 2004 dialogue among pharmacy leaders together and also served as a Global Health Consultant on the GHAIN project.

Others whom I have been privileged to collaborate with include:
- Dr. Anthony Wutoh, provost and chief academic officer at Howard University who wrote a section of one of the TrainPharm manuals on HIV/AIDS.
- Dr. Douglas Keene, vice president of Management Sciences for Health, who is now retired.
- Dr. Terri Moore, who previously worked at the U.S. Department of Health and Human Services and is now the senior director of academic services at the American Association of Colleges of Pharmacy.
- Dr. Donna McCree, Associate Director for Health Equity/ Division of HIV/AIDS Prevention, Center for Disease Control and Prevention

These colleagues showed little hesitation when opportunities arose to join forces on this path of public health. Further, there have been many, many young pharmacists who have sought my advice. In 1992, I participated in a symposium held by the Cameroon Students Association in the United States. Nicholas Vega, the national president at the time, wrote me a letter afterwards, stating:

Your presentation was enlightening and a surprise to many Cameroonians. Because we consider health care an important issue in Cameroon, we the Cameroon Students in the United

States would like to invite you once more for another presentation on health care in our next symposium.

My career has taken me across the United States as well as internationally. Throughout the years, I have been licensed as a pharmacist in five states – New York, my home state; Pennsylvania, where I went to school; Delaware, where I spent a summer developing an organization called Pharmacists Access to Health Care (PATH), which advocated for pharmacists being frontline health workers; California, where I did most of my traditional work as a pharmacist; and Arkansas, where my husband and I once considered relocating. As I write in 2020, all my licenses are now officially inactive.

But pharmacy has also allowed me to expand the topic of global health in the Pharmacy conversation. In 2007, Dean David Knapp of the University of Maryland School of Pharmacy asked that I be their commencement speaker. My theme was, "Going Forth into the Global Marketplace." I encouraged the students to look beyond working in the U.S. If they had the chance, I advised them to look for opportunities to work with colleagues in other countries. I recommended that they explore the world and their ability to make a difference globally. I also shared with the students anecdotes from my experiences abroad, including some the interesting minutiae of my work. For instance, because I did so much official, international travel, I wound up having plural passports over the years. I sometimes needed multiple passports during the same time period, such as when I traveled for the U.S. Department of State. At one time, I had two passports – one of them could only be used to travel to or transit through South Africa in the days of apartheid.

When I think back on my career, I am reminded of a speech I gave at Purdue University while I worked at APhA in which I talked about letting your difference make a difference. In the speech, I acknowledged that Black folks are treated differently within the context of American society, but we can make a difference in this world wherever we are.

I also think about the change that can happen from consulting with global colleagues intellectually instead of "parachuting" in as an expert.

The impact of my work was not just professional, but also personal. When I worked in many countries, I was not a part of their culture, and I had to do my best not to inadvertently buy into cultural oppression, even as I worked as a technical consultant.

Yet, I would often be asked questions about my own experience as an African American. I would be asked how Black Americans survived Jim Crow laws and general discrimination. I was able to connect with people in the countries I visited by relating my experiences as an African American to the experience that they suffered under colonization or other forms of oppression.

And, what happened to my food allergies and eczema? It restricted my choice of foods in many places to which I traveled, which caused many to question if I just did not want to have a meal with them or if I was really allergic. I still have my allergies and eczema; they have progressed, but in no way have they stopped me from my purpose – sharing what I have learned at the junction of pharmacy and public health. In all, it is proof positive that God protected me throughout all my journeys. There was only one occasion that I fell ill, and it was due to a cold, not an allergic reaction or a flare-up of eczema.

I will always cherish the connections I made across the world during my career. I am grateful to have played a small role in helping change the way pharmacists are able to serve across the globe.

Being a pharmacist with training in public health has given me an opportunity to realize my purpose in serving underserved communities around the world. It has allowed me to push past limitations and help others see that pharmacists could play an invaluable role in the healthcare system. I am appreciative of the opportunities I have had to contribute to better health care for all through "stick-to-it-tive-ness," spirituality, and commitment. I trust that I have answered the question of "what did you do."

Now to those pharmacists who come after me, it is your turn, dear reader, dear student, to take up the mantle, gather a few risks, map out a path, or "let your difference make a difference," to leave your footprint in the sands of time. Show what pharmacists can do!

Epilogue

The Planting of Seeds Precedes the Harvest

On April 22, 2020, USAID posted a PEPFAR Solution strategic information document written under the Howard University/FHI 360 partnership: (https://www.pepfarsolutions.org/solutions/2020/4/21/leveraging-private-pharmacists-to-expand-art-distribution-promote-adherence-and-mobilize-resources accessed 5/1/2020). The identified Solution, which pointed to the use of private pharmacists of Nigeria to expand ART services, is an impactful, data-driven implementing experience that can serve as a "how-to" guide for others.

PEPFAR leverages the power of partnerships across multiple sectors to increase its impact and advance sustainability. One such partnership is the Howard University/FHI360 partnership with USAID which has focused on Pharmacist and Pharmacy since 2004. This has resulted in a designated PEPFAR SOLUTION.

PEPFAR is the largest commitment by any nation to address a single disease in history. Through the compassion and generosity of the American people, PEPFAR has saved and improved millions of lives, accelerating progress toward controlling and ultimately ending the AIDS epidemic as a public health threat. (https://www.state.gov/pepfar/ accessed 9/01/20).

The PEPFAR Solutions Platform is a user-friendly space to access and share data-driven implementation practices across HIV programmatic areas and geographic regions, to drive achievement of HIV epidemic control. (https://pepfarsolutions.squarespace.com/epidemic-control ac cessed 5/1/2020)

This chronicle has highlighted some seeds planted to promote the full engagement of pharmacists and pharmacies. An early seed was the 1985 Pharmaceuticals in Health Assistance (a USAID guidance document), which focused on access to drugs – including wider use of private pharmacists and pharmacies.

A second seed was the collaboration with WAPF and the production of the AWAP report, a portion of which gives the 2001 Accra Recommendation (named after the city in which the ending conference was held), and reads:

- *The community **pharmacist** is a recognized health professional contributing to a favorable health outcome; and*
- *The community **pharmacy** is a patient contact site, a health service outlet close to the population which can be a fulcrum for improved health status of a community.*

A third seed was the GHAIN project in 2004, for it laid the vision of a focused inclusion of a Pharmacy and pharmacists' component in the flagship PEPFAR project in Nigeria.

Even though in this chronicle many seeds are identified, the flowering of a focus on pharmacists as contributing frontline health workers in a PEPFAR solutions platform confirms that harvesting has come in a new season.

At the close of the 2004 Dialogue, Dr. Gloria Niemeyer Francke, renowned Remington Medalist and Pharmacist Extraordinaire, said that she hoped all attendees, especially pharmacist and pharmacy leaders, would go forth as advocates continuing a dialogue to ensure that the seeds planted that day would come forth as "big apples."

Community Pharmacists in Nigeria, under the leadership of Howard University Global Initiative director, Dr. Dorothy Oqua, as a part of the USAID-funded partnership with FHI360, are demonstrating significant frontline contribution to improved health in their community.

And so, seed planting continues into the next season....

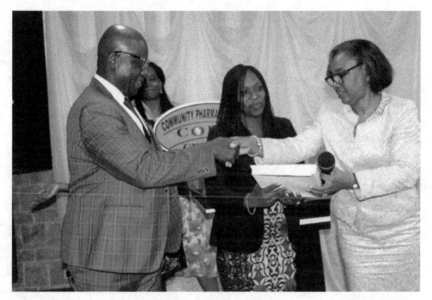

Dr. Dorothy Oqua, Country Director, HUGIN (R), presenting an award plaque to Pharmacist Ike Onyechi, Managing Director, Alpha Pharmacy Nigeria Limited, at an event.

(https://www.pharmanewsonline.com/applause-as-17-pharmacies-bag-copa-awards/ accessed 4/25/2020)

Acronyms

A&S	Abraham & Straus
ABCOTS	American Baptist Churches of the South
ACLU	American Civil Liberties Union
AJHP	American Journal of Health-Systems Pharmacists
APED	Action Program on Essential Drugs
APhA	American Pharmaceutical Association
APHA	American Public Health Association
ASHP	American Society of Health-System Pharmacists
AWAP	Anglophone West Africa Pharmaceutical Federation
CDC	Centers for Disease Control and Prevention
CLAPA	Central Los Angeles Pharmaceutical Association
DART	Drew Ambulatory Care Review Team
DHEW/HSA	Department of Health Education & Welfare, Health Services Administration
DRC	Democratic Republic of the Congo
FAA	Federal Aviation Administration
FAMU	Florida Agriculture and Mechanical University
FDA	Food and Drug Administration
FHI	Family Health International
FOF	Family of the Future
FSI	Foreign Service Institute
GHAIN	Global HIV/AIDS Initiative Nigeria
HBCU	Historically Black College/University
HU	Howard University
HUCE	Howard University Continuing Education
HUGIN	Howard University Global Initiative in Nigeria
ICASA	International Conference on AIDS and STD in Africa

IHI	International Health Institute
IPA	Intergovernmental Personnel Action
N.G.O.S.	Non-Governmental Organizations
NAFDAC	National Agency for Food and Drug Control
NIPRD	Nigerian Institute of Pharmaceutical Research and Development
NPhA	National Pharmaceutical Association
OEO	Office of Economic Opportunity
OIP	Office of International Programs
PACE	Pharmacists and Continuing Education
PATH	Program for Appropriate Technology in Health
PCN	Pharmacists Council of Nigeria
PEPFAR	U.S. President's Emergency Plan for Aids Relief
PIET	Program for International Education and Training
PSN	Pharmaceutical Society of Nigeria
ROADS	Regional Outreach Addressing AIDS through Development Strategies
S.E.S.A.	Santé De L'Enfant du Sud et Adamaoua
SAPhA	Student American Pharmaceutical Association
SCHARP	Sustaining Comprehensive HIV/AIDS Response through Partnership
SECON	Systems Evaluation of Care Consultants
SIDHAS	Strengthening Integrated Delivery of HIV/AIDS Services
TB	Tuberculosis
TSU	Texas Southern University
UCLA	University of California Los Angeles
UNIKIN	University of Kinshasa
USAID	United States Agency of International Development
USC	University of Southern California
USP	United States Pharmacopeia
USP/DI	United States Pharmacopeial Drug Information
USPC	United States Pharmacopeial Convention
WAPF	West African Pharmaceutical Federation
WASP	White Anglo-Saxon Protestant
WHO	World Health Organization

Bibliography

American Public Health Association (APHA). 2006. *The Role of the Pharmacist in Public Health.* Policy Number 200614, Washington, DC: APHA.

American Public Health Association (APHA). 1981. *The Role of the Pharmacist in Public Health.* Policy Statement 8024, Washington, DC: APHA.

American Society of Health-System Pharmacists. 1981. "Statement on the Role of Health-System Pharmacists in Public Health." *American Journal of Health-System Pharmacists (AJHP).*

Cain, Rosalyn M. December 1970. "New Dimensions in Practice: The Neighborhood Health Center Pharmacy." *American Journal of Pharmaceutical Education* Vol 14.

Cain, Rosalyn M., and Joel Kahn. 1971. "The Pharmacist As a Member of the Health Team." *American Journal of Public Health* 2223-8.

FHI360, and Howard University. 2012. *GHAIN Support To HIV-Related Pharmaceutical Servcices In Nigeria.* End of Project Monograph, Alexandria, VA: United States Agency for International Development (USAID); FHI360.

International Health Institute. 1992. *Project S.E.S.A. (Santé De L'Enfant du Sud et Adamaoua) Child Health in South and Adamaoua Provinces in Cameroon.* Project Report, Los Angeles, CA: Charles R. Drew University of Medicine and Science.

Kahn, Joel, Rosalyn M. Cain, and Sydney P. Galloway. 1970. "Pharmacy in Poverty Areas; A Literature Search." *Journal of the American Pharmaceutical Association* 466-468.

King, Rosalyn C, and Dorothy Oqua. 2019. "Dynamic Relationship Between Education, Regulation and Practice: Case Studies and Examples - Nigeria." *Encyclopedia of Pharmacy Practice and Clinical Pharmacy.* Edited by Zaheer-Ud-Din Baber. Compiled by Michael J Rouse and Lina R Bader. Amsterdam: Elsevier - Academic Press. doi:10.1016/B978-0-12-812735-3.00133-3.

King, Rosalyn C, and Felicia Loghin. 2019. "Dynamic Relationship Between Education, Regulation and Practice: Case Studies and Examples - Romania." *Encyclopedia of Pharmacy Practice and and Clinical Pharmacy.* Edited by Zaher-Ud-Din Babar. Compiled by Michael J Rouse and Lina R Bader. Amsterdam: Elsevier- Academic Pres. doi:10.1016. B978-0-12-812735-3.013-3.

King, Rosalyn C. 1988. *Guidance for Developing the Project's Propharmacy System in Adamoua and South Provinces as a Key to Primary Health Care Financing & Sustainability.* Project Guidance, Los Angeles, CA: Charles R. Drew University.

King, Rosalyn C. 1981. *Providing Basic Medicines in Rural Primary Health Care Projects in Africa: Technical Guidelines.* Consultant Report, Washington, D.C.: United States Agency for International Development (USAID).

King, Rosalyn C. 1981. *The Provision of Pharmaceuticals in Selected Primary Health Care Projects in Africa: Report of a Survey.* Survey Report, Washington, D.C.: United States Agency for International Development (USAID).

Robinson, Ira C., King, Rosalyn C. 1978. "Black Pharmacists in the U.S. and How Their Status is Changing." *American Druggist* 13-16.

Sardell, Alice. 1988. *The U.S. Experiment in Social Medicine: The Community Health Center Progam 1965-1986.* Pittsburgh, PA: University of Pittsburgh Press.

Unitd States Agency for International Development. 2008. *Transport Corridor Program Mid-Term Assessment.* Evaluation Team Report, Washington, DC: United States Agency for International Development.

United States Agency for International Development; Essential Drugs Committee. 1985. *Program Guidance Paper on Pharmaceuticals in Health Assistance.* Committee Chair's Report, Washington, D.C.: United States Agency for International Development (USAID), Office of Health and Population.

2017. "www.washingtonpost.com." October 18. Accessed February 5, 2020. https://www.washingtonpost.com/lifestyle/style/the-curious-story-of-the-malls-lone-privately-owned-plot/2017/10/18/9d894632-b27e-11e7-9e58-e6288544af98_story.html

Index

CPSIA information can be obtained
at www.ICGtesting.com
Printed in the USA
LVHW082037210521
688188LV00002B/175